Evaluating Psychometric Properties of Spanish Neuropsychological Tests for Older Latinos

United States Consortium of Aging
Dementia & Latino Studies (CADLAS)

Evaluating Psychometric Properties of Spanish Neuropsychological Tests for Older Latinos

Evaluating Psychometric Properties of Spanish Neuropsychological Tests for Older Latinos

ISBN-13: 978-1-951166-48-9 (Print)
ISBN-13: 978-1-951166-49-6 (eBook)

Cover Design: Falcone Creative Design, LLC, Octal Productions, LLC
Book Design: Dianne Russell, Octal Productions, LLC
Book Production: Octal Productions, LLC
Director: Jane Pimental, Division of Professional and Public Education
Program Manager: Heather Carillo, MGH Psychiatry Academy
Administrative Coordinator: Alexandra D. Fowler, MGH Psychiatry Academy
Printing and Binding: RP Graphics
This book is printed on acid-free paper.

About the Author

Established in 2022, the U.S. Consortium of Aging, Dementia & Latino Studies (CADLAS) is a national collaborative research network committed to advancing knowledge of aging, Alzheimer's disease, and related dementias in U.S. Latino populations. By fostering interdisciplinary collaboration, the Consortium aims to accelerate scientific discovery, strengthen the development and validation of biomarkers and diagnostic tools, and improve strategies for prevention, treatment and care. CADLAS organizes its work across four core areas: 1) cognition and assessment; 2) genomics and biomarkers; 3) recruitment and clinical trials; and 4) dementia care and psychosocial interventions. Through these integrated efforts, the Consortium aims to reduce health disparities and promote more equitable, culturally responsive approaches to dementia research and clinical practice.

This volume was developed by the CADLAS Cognition and Assessment Special Interest Group to fill critical gaps in the validation of cognitive and clinical assessment tools for Spanish-speaking older adults and to provide a framework for more culturally and linguistically appropriate evaluation of cognitive functioning in older Latinos.

About the Author

Dedication

This book is dedicated to the Latino community in the United States—particularly to older Latinos, whose lived experiences, resilience, and cultural richness continue to shape our understanding of cognitive health and aging. Your participation in research and your trust in the scientific and clinical communities have been essential to advancing more accurate, equitable, and culturally responsive neuropsychological assessment. We hope this work contributes to improved recognition, diagnosis, and care that honor your language and cultural identity.

Acknowledgements

The contributing authors gratefully acknowledge all members of the U.S. Consortium of Aging, Dementia & Latino Studies (CADLAS) for their unwavering dedication to improving the lives of older Latinos affected by Alzheimer's disease and related dementias. We extend our sincere thanks not only for essential work each member undertakes in their respective roles, but also for the additional time, energy, and commitment devoted to advancing the Consortium's mission. These collective efforts reflect the power of collaboration and a shared commitment to meaningful change.

We also honor the Latino individuals and families living with dementia and express our deepest gratitude to those who have participated in research studies. Your generosity and trust are instrumental in advancing scientific understanding of these diseases and moving us closer to a future in which aging does not mean the loss of cognitive function, dignity, or independence.

Together, we stand united in the fight against dementia.

How This Book Is Organized

The book is organized to move from foundational concepts through clinical practice to research:

1. **Foundations of psychometrics and cultural considerations:** Key principles of test design, reliability, validity, and fairness.
2. **Domains of neuropsychological function:** Discussion of intelligence, memory, attention, processing speed, executive function, language, visuospatial abilities, and motor skills.
3. **Spanish-language test review:** Examination of psychometric properties and normative data for tests developed in the U.S., Latin America, and Spain, with particular emphasis on norms that control for educational level.
4. **Assessment of bilingualism, cultural factors, acculturation, and educational experience:** These factors significantly influence test performance and interpretation. Incorporating them into the evaluation process leads to more accurate and culturally appropriate clinical diagnoses.
5. **Clinical and research applications:** Practical guidance for selecting tests, administering them appropriately, and applying results to diagnosis and research.
6. **Future directions:** Emerging trends in culturally informed neuropsychological testing, including digital tools, biomarkers, and global collaborations.

By bringing together research, practice, and cultural considerations, this book aims to advance the accuracy, equity, and impact of neuropsychological assessment on older, Spanish-speaking Latino/Hispanic adults, ultimately improving brain health outcomes across diverse communities.

Table of Contents

Contributors

Mónica Rosselli, PhD
Professor and Neuropsychologist
Department of Psychology
Florida Atlantic University
Davie, Florida
1Florida Alzheimer's Disease Research Center
Miami, FL

Yakeel T. Quiroz, PhD
Clinical Neuropsychologist and Professor
Department of Psychiatry
Massachusetts General Hospital
Department of Psychological & Brain Sciences
Boston University
Boston, MA

Daniel G. Saldana, PhD
Clinical Neuropsychologist
Instructor of Psychology
Department of Psychiatry
Massachusetts General Hospital
Boston, MA

Cynthia Abinader, PsyD
Postdoctoral Fellow
Department of Neurology
Hospital of the University of Pennsylvania
Philadelphia, PA

Paula A. Aduen, PhD
Neuropsychologist
Assistant Professor of Psychology
Department of Psychiatry and Psychology
Mayo Clinic
Jacksonville, FL

Jordana Breton, MA
Graduate Student Fellow
The University of Texas
Austin, TX

Flavio Carhuavilca, BA
Post-Baccalaureate Student
Department of Psychology
Florida Atlantic University
Davie, FL

Carmen I. Carrión, PsyD
Neuropsychologist
Associate Professor of Neurology
Yale School of Medicine
New Haven, CT

Rosie E. Curiel, PsyD
Neuropsychologist and Professor
Department of Psychiatry and Behavioral Sciences at the University of Miami Miller School of Medicine
1Florida Alzheimer's Disease Research Center
Miami, FL

Malyorie Garcia-Diaz, PsyD
Postdoctoral Fellow
Wien Center for Alzheimer's Disease and Memory
Mount Sinai Medical Center, and Florida ADRC
Miami, FL

Zoraida C. Garcia, BSA
Project Manager
University of Texas
Austin, TX

Averi Giudicessi, MS
PhD Student
Department of Psychological and Brain Science
Boston University
Boston, MA

Yaimara Gonzalez Pineiro, BS
Clinical Research Associate
Wein Center for Alzheimer's Disease
Memory Disorders at Mount Sinai
Medical Center
Alzheimer's Disease Research Center
Miami, FL

Alicia Goytizolo, MA
Doctoral Student
Department of Psychology
Florida Atlantic University
Boca Raton, FL

Melissa Lamar, PhD
Professor and Clinical Neuropsychologist
Rush Alzheimer's Disease Center &
Department of Psychiatry and
Behavioral Sciences
Rush University Medical Center
Chicago, IL

Merike Lang, PhD
Postdoctoral Fellow
Department of Psychology
Florida Atlantic University
Davie, FL

Tatiana Mercedes, MS, EdM, MA
Clinical Psychology Doctoral Student
Ponce Health Sciences University
Ponce, PR

Ambar Perez Lao, BA
Doctoral Candidate
Department of Clinical and
Health Psychology University of Florida
Gainesville, FL

Alexandra Ortega, PsyD
Research Assistant Professor
Department of Psychiatry and
Behavioral Sciences at the University of
Miami Miller School of Medicine
Miami, FL

Katya Rascovsky, PhD
Associate Professor
Department of Neurology and Penn
Frontotemporal Degeneration Center
University of Pennsylvania
Perelman School of Medicine
Philadelphia, PA

Nathan Raymond Ramirez, PsyD
Neuropsychologist
Aptiva Health, Concussion &
Sports Medicine Institute
Louisville, KY

Glariangeliz Tapia-Nazario, MS
Clinical Psychology Pre-Doctoral Intern
Ponce Health Sciences University
Ponce, PR

Idaly Velez Uribe, PhD
Research Manager
Wien Center for Alzheimer's Disease and
Memory Disorders
Mount Sinai Medical Center
Miami, FL

Melanie Ventura, PsyD
Clinical Neuropsychology Fellow
Department of Neurology
University of Virginia School of Medicine
Charlottesville, VA

Clara Vila-Castelar, PhD
Assistant Professor
Washington University
St. Louis, MO

Zvinka Z. Zlatar, PhD
Associate Professor
Department of Psychiatry
University of California
San Diego, CA

Introduction

Alzheimer's disease (AD) and related dementias represent one of the most pressing health challenges of our time, with disproportionate impact on Latino/Hispanic communities in the United States (U.S.). Approximately 13% of Latinos/Hispanics aged 65 and older live with AD or another form of dementia—significantly higher than the 10% prevalence among older non-Latino white adults, underscoring a clear health disparity (Matthews et al, 2019; Quiroz et al, 2022). An accurate diagnosis of mild cognitive impairment (MCI) and dementia relies on cognitive and functional test performance, making the psychometric properties of these assessments critical (Burke et al, 2019). While results of neuroimaging and blood tests may help to establish an etiology, the neuropsychological evaluation is important for diagnosis, clinical staging, and characterization of the clinical syndrome.

Previous reviews have examined the availability of normative data and assessment tools for Spanish-speaking and Latino/Hispanic populations (Morlett Paredes et al, 2021). More recently, Perez-Lao et al. (2025) conducted a systematic review that examined normative data for Spanish speakers across the U.S., Spain, and Latin America. The review systematically analyzed literature retrieved from six major databases to characterize the current landscape of normative data spanning pediatric to geriatric age groups. Seventy-five peer-reviewed studies met the inclusion criteria and were synthesized to provide a summary of norms limited to peer-reviewed publications.

This book was developed to build upon prior work and to address existing gaps in the validation of cognitive and clinical assessments for Spanish-speaking older adults. The Cognition and Assessment Special Interest Group of the U.S. Consortium of Aging, Dementia, and Latino Studies (CADLAS, https://cadlas.org/) conducted a comprehensive review of available Spanish-language assessment instruments and offered recommendations for their application in clinical and research settings. Expanding on that foundation, the present volume examines the psychometric properties and normative methodologies of assessments developed in the U.S., Latin America, and Spain for adults aged 55 and older, highlighting their respective strengths and limitations (see Table on page 132).

Who Should Read This Book?

This book is designed for clinicians, neuropsychologists, neurologists, geriatricians, researchers, students, and other healthcare professionals interested in culturally informed neuropsychological assessment. Families, caregivers, and community advocates may also find value in understanding why culturally and linguistically appropriate testing matters in diagnosis and care.

What Does Knowledge of Psychometrics Offer?

Psychometrics provides a framework for evaluating the validity, reliability, and fairness of neuropsychological tests. Understanding psychometric principles allows clinicians to determine whether a test meaningfully measures cognitive function across cultural and linguistic groups, and whether test scores can guide accurate diagnoses, treatment planning, and research conclusions.

Where and When Should Neuropsychological Testing Be Conducted?

Neuropsychological testing can be conducted in hospitals, memory clinics, private practices, and research settings. Testing should be considered whenever individuals present with memory or other cognitive complaints (e.g., language problems or visuospatial changes), functional decline, or behavioral changes that raise concerns for neurological changes. It also plays a role in longitudinal care, monitoring disease progression, and evaluating treatment efficacy.

Why Is Neuropsychological Testing Necessary?

Accurate assessment is fundamental to establishing a diagnosis, differentiating among types of dementia, and guiding further evaluation. Without culturally sensitive testing, misdiagnosis is more likely, which can delay appropriate care, treatment, and support for patients and families.

How Is Neuropsychological Testing Conducted?

Neuropsychological testing can range from brief screening tools that take 10–30 minutes to comprehensive batteries requiring several hours. Tests are administered by trained professionals, often involving tasks that measure memory, attention, language, problem-solving, visuospatial skills, motor coordination, and processing speed.

FOUNDATIONS OF PSYCHOMETRICS AND CULTURAL CONSIDERATIONS

Neuropsychological Measures

Reviewing neuropsychological measures and evaluating normative studies requires close attention to psychometric properties that shape test construction. A central concept is reliability, which reflects the extent to which individual differences in test scores represent true differences in the construct being measured rather than chance or error (Ahmed and Ishtiaq, 2021). Reliability in normative studies is usually expressed as a coefficient between 0 and 1.0, with values nearer to 1 indicating greater stability (Field, 2024). According to Stucky et al. (2020), common forms relevant to neuropsychological instruments include the following:

- Test–retest reliability (stability of scores across administrations)
- Alternate forms reliability (consistency across test versions)
- Split-half reliability (internal consistency)
- Inter-item reliability (consistency among items within a construct)
- Interrater reliability (agreement between independent raters)

Equally important is validity, or the degree to which a measure actually captures what it is intended to assess (Ahmed and Ishtiaq, 2021). According to Stucky et al. (2020), types of validity include the following:

- Content validity (how well a measure represents the domain of interest)
- Predictive validity (how well test scores forecast performance on a criterion, such as SAT scores predicting college outcomes)
- Concurrent validity (correspondence with an established measure)
- Construct validity (the extent to which the instrument reflects the underlying psychological trait)

Ensuring accurate and equitable neuropsychological assessment in Hispanic/Latino populations demands attention not only to reliability and validity but also to cultural and linguistic context. Historically, test development and large-scale normative studies have been rooted in WEIRD populations (Western, educated, industrialized, rich, and democratic) (Fernandez, 2019; Henrich, Heine, and Norenzayan, 2010). To enhance inclusivity, developers must consider factors such as literacy levels, educational quality, cultural frameworks, and how these interact with Western psychological constructs. Language structure also matters, since phonological, syntactic, and morphological features differ across languages and can shape test performance (Gasquoine et al, 2007; Marks et al, 2023; Muroya et al, 2017). Consideration of these aforementioned factors helps to improve test fairness and work toward limiting misdiagnosis, improving accurate estimation of cognitive and behavioral functioning, and increasing equitable access to assessment and treatment.

DOMAINS OF THE NEUROPSYCHOLOGICAL FUNCTION

Neuropsychological assessments characterize the severity and pattern of cognitive and behavioral impairments, offering insight into the structural and functional integrity of the brain. Using standardized measures, clinicians evaluate domains including attention, memory, language, processing speed, visuospatial skills, and executive functions (Lezak et al, 2012).

Brief cognitive screening tools provide a quick estimate of cognitive functioning and help identify patients who may require more comprehensive evaluation. Their usefulness, however, is tempered by variable sensitivity and susceptibility to demographic influences. For example, highly educated individuals may perform within the normal range despite subtle deficits, while those with fewer years of education, different primary languages, or distinct cultural backgrounds may be misclassified as impaired. These limitations highlight the importance of interpreting screening results within the broader clinical and demographic context.

Interpretation requires appropriate normative data and consideration of premorbid ability since most cognitive tasks rely on multiple processes and cannot independently distinguish between dementia syndromes. Instead, the full cognitive profile, the chronology of deficits, and test selection are essential to differential diagnosis.

Neuropsychological evaluations serve multiple purposes in the assessment and management of dementia. They are particularly valuable for differential diagnosis, helping to distinguish normal aging from mild cognitive impairment (MCI), to separate neurodegenerative disorders from potentially reversible causes of cognitive complaints such as depression, and to characterize dementia syndromes to inform etiology (for example, differentiating Alzheimer's disease from Frontotemporal dementia). These assessments also support the longitudinal tracking of progression, providing a baseline against which changes over time can be measured and allowing clinicians to monitor the effects of medications or behavioral interventions. Importantly, impairments detected through neuropsychological testing can act as predictive biomarkers, offering early indications of conversion from MCI to Alzheimer's disease or other dementias.

In addition to diagnosis and prognosis, neuropsychological evaluations shed light on functional abilities, identifying specific areas of daily living where support may be needed, such as remembering appointments or managing medications. This information helps guide intervention strategies aimed at maintaining independence, which may include referrals to speech therapy, structured use of calendars or day planners, or the introduction of assistive technologies. They also play a role in assessing competence, providing objective data to aid families and clinicians in decisions about driving, as well as medical, financial, or legal decision-making capacity.

Finally, these evaluations contribute to research, where quantifying cognition and behavior enables correlations with structural and functional brain imaging, deepening understanding of the neural networks underlying different functions. Neuropsychological tests also serve as sensitive outcome measures in clinical trials, particularly for assessing the efficacy of disease-modifying therapies.

A formal neuropsychological assessment for dementia will usually evaluate the following domains (Rascovsky, 2016):

- **Attention and concentration:** Attention and concentration are necessary for adequate performance on any cognitive task. Attention and working memory are often assessed with forward and backward digit span, as well as tasks of vigilance and sustained attention. Fluctuating attention is characteristic of dementia with Lewy bodies (DLB), though it can be difficult to capture in a single evaluation.
- **Processing speed:** Processing speed is typically measured with timed tasks such as the Trail Making Test or Wechsler Adult Intelligence Scale (WAIS) Symbol Search. Slowed performance is commonly associated with disruption of fronto-subcortical circuits, as seen in Parkinson's disease (Sawamoto et al, 2002), Progressive Supranuclear Palsy (Kobylecki et al, 2015), and small-vessel vascular disease (Prins et al, 2005).
- **Memory:** Memory profiles are highly informative for differential diagnosis. Memory is broadly classified as declarative/explicit (conscious recollection of facts and events) and non-declarative/implicit (skills and procedures). Declarative memory is further divided into episodic memory, which refers to the recall of personal experiences, and semantic memory, which reflects knowledge of facts and concepts. Memory assessments probe encoding (ability to consolidate new information), retention (ability to retain this information over time), and retrieval (ability to recall information after a delay or interference) processes using word lists, story recall, or figure reproduction. Episodic memory impairment, particularly in learning and retention, is characteristic of Alzheimer's disease and amnestic MCI.

- **Language:** Neuropsychological testing provides detailed language profiles that aid diagnosis and guide interventions. Common assessments include spontaneous speech, naming (Boston Naming Test, Multilingual Naming Test), semantic knowledge, grammar (sentence-picture matching), reading, and repetition. Such profiles are especially valuable in differentiating primary progressive aphasia (PPA) variants. Non-fluent/agrammatic PPA presents with halting, agrammatic speech but preserved single-word comprehension and object knowledge. Semantic variant PPA features fluent but empty speech, anomia, and impaired word meaning. The logopenic variant, often associated with Alzheimer's disease and easily confused with the other forms, is marked by severe anomia and sentence repetition deficits despite intact motor speech, grammar, and basic comprehension.
- **Visuospatial and constructional tests** evaluate perception and reproduction of visual stimuli (e.g., block design, complex figure copy), with disproportionate visuospatial impairment often seen in dementia with Lewy bodies or posterior cortical atrophy.
- **Executive functions** are measured through tasks of planning, abstraction, mental flexibility, and inhibition (e.g., verbal fluency, Stroop, Trail Making Test, or Wisconsin Card Sorting Test). Prominent dysexecutive errors, such as perseveration or poor organization, are especially helpful in identifying frontotemporal syndromes.
- **Mood and behavior:** Self-report measures of mood and behavior, such as the Geriatric Depression Scale, can be used to evaluate symptoms of depression and anxiety. In dementia, however, limited insight often reduces the reliability of self-report, so clinicians frequently rely on informant-based behavioral scales. These instruments assess a range of neuropsychiatric symptoms, including hallucinations, delusions, disinhibition, apathy, and agitation. Widely used tools include the Neuropsychiatric Inventory, the Frontal Behavioral Inventory, and the Cambridge Behavioral Inventory.

Beyond diagnosis, neuropsychological assessments provide a baseline for monitoring disease progression, guide interventions to support independence (e.g., daily functioning strategies or therapy referrals), and inform judgments about driving or financial or medical decision-making capacity. They also serve as sensitive outcome measures in clinical research and clinical trials, and allow mapping of cognitive deficits onto underlying neural networks.

SPANISH-LANGUAGE TEST NORMALIZATION PROGRAMS

Methodology of Neuropsychological Test Normalization Programs in the United States, Latin America, and Spain

Developing culturally and linguistically appropriate neuropsychological norms is essential for accurately assessing Spanish-speaking populations, given their diverse educational, sociocultural, and immigration backgrounds. A number of large-scale normative efforts have been conducted across the United States, Latin America, and Spain, each using distinct sampling strategies, inclusion criteria, and analytic approaches to capture variation in demographic and linguistic factors. Below, we summarize key studies that have generated norms for Spanish-speaking adults, including U.S.-based initiatives (e.g., TMAANS, NP-NUMBRS, and UDS-NB3), multi-country projects in Latin America, population-based efforts in Colombia, and the NEURONORMA study in Spain. Together, these projects highlight both the progress and the persistent gaps in developing normative data for Spanish-speaking populations.

United States of America

Texas Mexican American Adult Normative Studies

TMAANS norms are based on 797 Mexican American adults aged 40+, assessed in their preferred language (Spanish: n = 412) by bilingual psychometrists (O'Bryant et al, 2018). Participants came from three cohorts:

- The Texas Alzheimer's Research & Care Consortium (TARCC; adults 50+ with normal cognition, MCI, or probable AD)
- The Health and Aging Brain Among Latino Elders (HABLE; community-based, n = 322, mostly women)
- FRONTIER (442 rural adults from three Texas counties)

Norms were derived from cognitively normal individuals (CDR = 0, consensus diagnosis) and stratified by demographic variables. Regression models tested age, gender, and education. Limitations include small subgroup sizes and no data on acculturation, years in the U.S., or age of English acquisition.

Neuropsychological Norms for the United States-Mexico Border Region in Spanish (NP-NUMBRS) Project

NP-NUMBRS included 254 Spanish-dominant adults (ages 18–60) from the California-Arizona border region, recruited across two cohorts (1998–2000 and 2006–2009). Exclusion criteria covered neurological, psychiatric, medical, or substance-related conditions. Trained bilingual psychometrists administered a comprehensive battery under strict quality protocols. Participants were classified as Spanish monolingual, English-dominant, or bilingual based on F-A-S fluency ratios, with education ranging from 0–20 years. Regression-based norms were generated. Limitations include modest sample size, restricted age range, and limited bilingualism data, making these norms most applicable to Spanish speakers from the U.S.-Mexico border (Cherner et al, 2021).

Uniform Data Set Neuropsychological Battery

The Uniform Data Set (UDS) of the National Institute on Aging Alzheimer's Disease Center Program includes a neuropsychological battery that has undergone three iterations:

- The UDSv2, neuropsychological battery was translated and adapted by researchers from Alzheimer's Disease Centers (ADCs) across the U.S. with expertise in the assessment of Spanish-speaking elderly. The resulting battery made provisions for variations among Spanish-speaking groups of different nationalities, socio-cultural, linguistic, and educational backgrounds (Acevedo et al, 2009).
- The UDSv2 neuropsychological battery included the MMSE, BNT-30, WMS-R Logical Memory (Story A), category fluency (animals and vegetables), TMT A&B, WAIS-R Digit Symbol, and WMS-R Digit Span. Benson et al. (2014) reported UDSv2 data from 276 cognitively normal Hispanic/Latino participants (CDR = 0) at 17 Alzheimer's Disease Research Centers, ADRCs (2007–2012), finding that age, sex, and education influenced scores; however, language proficiency was not measured.
- The UDS cognitive battery was updated in 2015 in coordination between the National Institute on Aging-appointed Clinical Task Force (CTF) and the National Alzheimer's Coordinating Center (NACC) (Weintraub et al, 2017). The UDSv3 includes the MoCA, Craft Story, Benson copy and recall, category and letter fluency, number span, TMT A&B, and MINT-32. Spanish translation of the UDSv3 involved preliminary translation and content review by expert clinicians, and pilot testing at three U.S. and four Latin American sites (Weintraub et al, 2018a).

Preliminary norms for English and Spanish-speaking U.S. Latino populations were provided by Marquine et al. (2023) and included 437 ADRC participants (191 Spanish speakers and 246 English speakers ages 50–94), with regression models examining demographic and language-of-testing effects.

The UDS neuropsychological battery has important strengths and some limitations. Its careful development and adaptation for Spanish-speaking populations improve cultural and linguistic validity, and the inclusion of widely used tests allows for a broad assessment of cognitive abilities. The creation of bilingual norms further supports its use across language groups. However, earlier versions did not assess language proficiency, and diverse Latino subgroups remain underrepresented, limiting generalizability. Demographic factors such as education, acculturation, and bilingualism also continue to influence performance, emphasizing the need for ongoing refinement and culturally sensitive norms.

Neuropsychological Norms for the Evaluation of Spanish-Speaking Adults in the United States (Rivera et al, 2024)

This study assessed 253 healthy Spanish-speaking adults (ages 18–80, M = 41) from eight U.S. states, mostly women. After excluding eight for missing data or low Spanish dominance, the final sample consisted of 245 participants who averaged 15.1 years of education (SD = 4.2; range 2–26), with 61.7% immigrating as adults. Acculturation and language dominance were measured with the Bidimensional Acculturation Scale for Hispanics (BAS) (Marin and Gamba, 1996) and the Bilingual Dominance Scale (Dunn and Fox Tree, 2009). Participants completed the following screening tests:

- The Mini-Mental State Examination (MMSE) >23
- The Patient Health Questionnaire-9 (PHQ) <10; Generalized Anxiety Disorder (GAD-7) <10
- A comprehensive neuropsychological battery spanning memory, attention, language, and executive function

Eligibility required ≥1 year of U.S. residency, ≥1 year of formal education, Spanish language dominance, and literacy in Spanish. Norms were generated using Bayesian regression models incorporating demographic predictors. Limitations include reliance on a novel Bayesian approach with high computational demands, unvalidated modeling of acculturation effects, and no measure of education quality.

Latin America

Ten Spanish Neuropsychological Tests in 11 Countries in Latin America

Normative data for 10 neuropsychological tests were collected from 3,977 healthy adults (ages 18–95) across 11 Latin American countries (Guardia-Olmos et al, 2015). Participants were native residents, primarily Spanish-speaking, with at least one year of education and no cognitive, neurological, psychiatric, or substance-related conditions.

Screening required Mini-Mental State Examination (MMSE) >23, Patient Health Questionnaire-9 (PHQ)-9 <10, and Generalized Anxiety Disorder (GAD-7) <10. A five-step procedure generated country-specific norms for the Rey-Osterrieth Complex Figure (ROCF), Stroop test, Modified Wisconsin Card Sorting Test (MWCST), Trail Making Test, Brief Test of Attention, phonemic and semantic fluency, Boston Naming Test, Symbol Digit Modalities Test, Hopkins Verbal Learning Test-Revised (HVLT-R), and Test of Memory Malingering (TOMM). These norms are valid only within their countries of origin. Limitations include the absence of bilingualism measures and other key sociodemographic variables, including acculturation, and not accounting for variability across countries. Education is characterized as less than or more than 12 years of education, which may exclude subtle influences otherwise captured by education as a continuous variable.

Colombian Alzheimer's Prevention Initiative Registry

Participants came from the Colombian Alzheimer's Prevention Initiative (API) registry of the Grupo de Neurociencias in Antioquia. Norms for the Consortium to Establish a Registry for Alzheimer's Disease (CERAD)–Colombia battery were developed using data from 2,673 cognitively unimpaired, non-carrier adults of the *PSEN1* E280A mutation (ages 18–86; mean education 8.9 years; 56.2% women). Age- and education-stratified norms were derived from means, SDs, and correlations, showing expected age-related declines in memory, fluency, and processing speed, with weaker effects of education (Torres et al, 2021). Limitations include an age-skewed sample (over half <30) and single-region recruitment, restricting generalizability.

Neuronorma

The Proyecto Neuronorma Colombia (NN-Co) (Montañés et al, 2020) established normative data from 438 cognitively normal adults ranging from aged 50–90 (mean education: 11 years; female 67.6%) and living in specific regions of Colombia, including Cundinamarca, Antioquia, Casanare, and Boyacá). This normative study included the same neuropsychological battery utilized in the original Neuronorma project (Peña-Casanova et al, 2012) with adaptation of measures and test order and standardization based on the Colombian population, with strengths including co-normalization. Age-, education-, and sex-stratified norms were derived from means, SDs, and correlations. Limitations include a predominantly female sample and a smaller sample size in >80-year-olds.

Spain

Neuronorma

The Neuronorma project (Peña-Casanova et al, 2009) established normative data from 356 cognitively intact Spanish adults (ages 49+) recruited from six regions of Spain, representing diverse sociocultural backgrounds. Inclusion required Spanish language fluency, basic literacy, independence in daily functioning (the Deterioration of Daily Living in

Dementia scale) (Teunisse, Derix, and van Crevel, 1991), and the absence of cognitive impairment (MMSE screening). Exclusion criteria covered central nervous system and systemic diseases linked to cognition, psychiatric illness, substance abuse, significant sensory deficits, and high scores on the Modified Ischemia Scale (Rosen et al, 1980). A broad neuropsychological battery, rigorously translated and adapted, was co-normed using an approach similar to the Mayo Clinic's older American normative studies, MOANS (Petersen et al, 1992), allowing cross-test comparisons. Strengths include regional sampling, standardized procedures, and co-normed scores; limitations include no analysis of bilingualism, absence of reliability indices, and limited generalizability to U.S. Spanish-speaking populations.

BRIEF MEASURES OF COGNITIVE SCREENING

Brief cognitive screening tools play an important role in clinical and research settings by enabling the early identification of cognitive impairment. They offer several advantages: they are efficient, typically taking less than 15 minutes to administer, and they provide a cognitive baseline that can be tracked over time. Additionally, they are accessible and low-cost, often usable by a range of trained professionals, and finally, they help guide decisions about whether a full neuropsychological evaluation is warranted. However, these tools also have notable limitations. Their scope is limited, assessing only broad cognitive domains and often missing more subtle or specific deficits. Cultural and educational biases can affect performance, particularly in individuals from diverse backgrounds, potentially leading to inaccurate results. These screenings lack diagnostic specificity, as they may suggest that something is wrong but cannot identify the underlying cause of impairment. Lastly, there is also a risk of false positives and negatives: high-functioning individuals with impairments may score within normal limits, while others may perform poorly for reasons unrelated to cognitive decline.

Importantly, the following brief cognitive screens are not a substitute for comprehensive assessment and should not be used in isolation to make significant clinical decisions.

The Mini-Mental State Examination (MMSE) has been the most widely used screening tool for cognitive impairment (Folstein, Folstein, and PR, 1975). Nonetheless, it has constraints: it does not assess abstraction or executive functions, and it is known to be influenced by socio-educational factors (Arevalo-Rodriguez et al, 2015).

Ostrosky-Solís et al. (2000) tested the sensitivity and specificity of the Spanish MMSE in 430 individuals aged 16–89 from Mexico and a group of 40 patients with dementia. Their educational levels ranged from zero years to having a college degree.

Two samples were independently studied. The first one included neurologically intact participants, and the second one consisted of patients with a clinical diagnosis of dementia. A total sample of 430 healthy participants ages 16–85. Inclusion criteria were (a) absence of dementia and (b) no history of neurological or psychiatric illness (e.g., cerebrovascular accidents, traumatic brain injury, epilepsy, or Parkinson's disease) according to clinical records and a neurological examination. All the participants were active and functionally independent. The sample was recruited from institutions for the elderly and people living in Mexico City and Colima. The second sample included 40 participants diagnosed with dementia. All the participants met the *DSM–IV* diagnostic criteria for dementia.

The effects of age and education were evaluated through analyses of variance (ANOVAs). The significance of $p < .001$ was established after the Bonferroni correction. Means and standard deviations according to age (three levels) and schooling (four levels) were obtained for the cognitively normal and the group with dementia. Specificity and sensitivity for a cutoff point of 23/24 were obtained. Receiver operating characteristic analyses for different cutoff values were further determined.

Rosselli et al. (2000) used the Spanish version of the MMSE in a Colombian population (N = 1611), including a high percentage of illiterate individuals. The sample was drawn from the five primary urban centers in Colombia: Bogotá, Medellín, Cali, Barranquilla, and Bucaramanga. Age was categorized into six groups (50–54, 55–59, 60–64, 65–69, 70–74, and 75 and older). Spearman's method was employed to establish a correlation matrix among the test components. Additionally, correlations were examined between the test components, total score, and the variables sex, education, and age. Pearson's correlations and linear regressions analyzed the relationship between continuous variables (total score, age, and education). ANOVAs assessed the contribution of each MMSE component to the total score, stratified by sex, education, and age variables. Finally, factor analysis was conducted on the 19 MMSE variables using the principal components method, chosen due to the mix of dichotomous and polychotomous variables present.

The 37-item version of the MMSE (MMSE-37) is an extended version of the original test for individuals with low education, which was adapted for diverse cultures. As part of the Neurological Disorders in Central Spain (NEDICES) study, Contador et al. (2016) presented normative data for >3,000 individuals from Spain aged 65–97. They stratified normative data according to age and education. All participants were defined as white, came from three clinics, and included unimpaired and impaired individuals. This revised version of the test incorporates several modifications to minimize the influence of education on test scores by simplifying specific tasks. For instance, this can be done by replacing the task of spelling "MUNDO" backward with a backward digit span task, introducing culturally-neutral items, such as visual sequencing (e.g., a man raising his hands), and broadening the scoring range to mitigate both floor and ceiling effects. The impact of sociodemographic factors (age, sex, and education) on MMSE-37 scores was assessed using Pearson's correlations and independent samples t-tests. Subsequently, a hierarchical regression was conducted to evaluate the individual contributions of these factors to MMSE-37 scores. Given the non-normal distribution of raw test scores, parametric statistics were validated using non-parametric equivalents (Spearman correlation and Mann-Whitney U test). Normative data were divided into nine overlapping age tables with midpoints at 66, 69, 72, 75, 78, 81, 84, 87, and 90 years using the technique of overlapping cell procedure.

Montreal Cognitive Assessment

The Montreal Cognitive Assessment (MoCA) is a cognitive screening tool that evaluates executive functions, attention, abstraction, memory, language, visuospatial skills, calculation, and orientation (Nasreddine et al, 2005). It has a maximum score of 30 points.

Delgado et al. (2019) validated the Spanish-language version of the Montreal Cognitive Assessment (MOCA-S) test in adults >60 years from Santiago de Chile. A total of 172 individuals were included: amnestic MCI (n = 24), non-amnestic MCI (n = 24), mild dementia (n = 20), and cognitively normal (n = 104). The discriminant validity of the MoCA-S was evaluated through three analyses:

- Comparisons of MoCA-S performance across groups, adjusting for age, sex, and education levels using ANCOVA and Bonferroni post hoc tests.
- Standardized mean differences, 95% confidence intervals, and Cohen's d effect sizes were calculated to quantify the extent of these differences.
- Receiver operating characteristic (ROC) curves were compared based on the area under the curve (AUC). A z statistic ≥1.5 was considered statistically significant.

Sensitivity, specificity, positive and negative predictive values, along with their 95% confidence intervals, were calculated. The Youden index guided the selection of the optimal cutoff point, prioritizing specificity to minimize false positives. Convergent validity between the MoCA-S and MMSE was assessed using Pearson correlation analysis. Internal consistency was evaluated using Cronbach's alpha, and reliability was examined using the Spearman correlation coefficient.

Aguilar-Navarro et al. (2018) validated the Spanish version of the MoCA in Mexico (MoCA-S), including 168 participants from a memory clinic in Mexico City: 59 were cognitively normal, 52 had MCI, and 57 had dementia (M_{age} = 76 ± 8.1). Spearman's correlation coefficient was employed to assess construct validity (convergence) by comparing results of the MoCA-S to the MMSE, standardized by education and age. ANOVAs examined sociodemographic differences and established criterion validity by testing the performance of the MoCA-S against a clinical assessment across three groups. Reliability was evaluated using test-retest reliability, estimating the intraclass correlation coefficient over a three-month interval. Internal consistency was determined using Cronbach's coefficient, with values considered very good if the score was >0.80, good between 0.70 and 0.80, moderate from 0.45 to 0.60, and poor if it was <0.45. Concordance was assessed by comparing results from each instrument with clinical diagnosis using the kappa coefficient, with an agreement ≥0.45 considered acceptable. ROC curves and the AUC were calculated to estimate sensitivity, specificity, positive predictive value (PPV), and negative predictive value (NPV) with 95% confidence intervals [95% CI].

Pereiro et al. (2017) administered the MoCA to 563 adult community members from Spain, aged 50–97. Four levels of education were considered (1–4, 5–8, 9–13, >13 years of formal schooling). The convergent validity was good, and the divergent validity was within the recommended range. Percentiles for age and educational level were calculated using regression coefficients and the standard deviation of the residual. Sex had a very small effect and was removed from the regression equation.

Strengths and Limitations: The MMSE and MoCA are among the most widely used screening tools for cognitive function, but both have important limitations. Their scores are strongly influenced by age and education, introducing cultural and educational bias (e.g., tasks such as spelling "world" backward). As a result, comparisons across individuals with different demographic backgrounds can be problematic. Both measures also have limited sensitivity: the MMSE may miss subtle impairments, especially in highly educated individuals, while the MoCA, though somewhat stronger in executive function assessment, can still show ceiling effects. Neither test provides a comprehensive evaluation of executive functions such as planning or problem-solving. In addition, repeated administrations may produce practice effects that inflate performance independent of cognitive change. Finally, MMSE norms are decades old and may not reflect the demographic diversity of current populations.

Evaluación Neuropsicológica Breve en Español

Evaluación Neuropsicológica Breve en Español (NEUROPSI) (Ostrosky-Solis et al, 1999) is a comprehensive yet brief neuropsychological screening tool for Spanish-speaking adults assessing nine domains (orientation, attention/concentration, language, memory, visuo-motor, executive functions, reading, writing, and calculation). Administration time is approximately 25–30 minutes.

The normative group included 800 cognitively intact Spanish-speaking monolingual volunteers from five Mexican cities (urban and rural: Mexico City, Colima, Toluca, Morelos, and Oaxaca) collected over four years. Participants were aged 16–85 (52% female). Age groups were divided into 16–30, 31–50, 51–65, and 66–85. Education ranged from 0–24 years, with four initial groups (illiterate, 1–4, 5–9, and 10–24 years). The highest bracket (10–24) was further divided into 10–12, 13–17, and 18–24. Norms were stratified by both age and education. Test-retest reliability over three months was .89, and interrater agreement ranged from .77 to 1.0. A later adaptation in Argentina (Querejeta et al, 2012) established age- and education-stratified norms for 656 participants, extending applicability beyond Mexico.

Strengths and Limitations: Strengths include a large and diverse normative sample and wide educational coverage. Limitations include a lack of psychometric indices beyond reliability (e.g., validity, sensitivity, and specificity), generalizability restricted to Mexican and Argentinian populations, and normative data capped at age 85.

Addenbrooke's Cognitive Examination—Revised/III (ACE-R/ACE-III in Spanish)

The Addenbrooke's Cognitive Examination (ACE) and its revised versions (ACE-R and ACE-III) are comprehensive cognitive screening tools designed to improve upon the MMSE by assessing five domains on a 100-point scale: attention/orientation, memory, language, fluency, and visuospatial skills, (Mioshi et al, 2006).

The Spanish ACE-R was validated in Argentina (Torralva et al, 2011), demonstrating excellent reliability ($\alpha = 0.89$, $\kappa = 0.98$) and strong diagnostic accuracy (97.5% sensitivity, 88.5% specificity) for dementia, outperforming the MMSE in distinguishing AD from behavioral variant Frontotemporal Dementia (bvFTD). The ACE-III was later validated in Spain (Matias-Guiu et al, 2015; Matias-Guiu et al, 2017), showing high internal consistency ($\alpha = 0.93$), strong reliability, and superior diagnostic accuracy, particularly in highly educated individuals; comprehensive normative data stratified by age, education, and gender were also provided. Additional validations include Argentina/Chile (Bruno et al, 2020), where the test distinguished AD from bvFTD with good reliability ($\alpha = 0.87$) and high classification accuracy, and Peru (Custodio et al, 2012), which used the Spanish ACE (predecessor to ACE-III) in healthy controls and patients with AD and FTD. The test showed strong internal consistency, high concurrent validity with the MMSE and ADAScog, and perfect diagnostic accuracy at a cut-off of 86 (100% sensitivity and specificity). These findings support its effectiveness for dementia screening in Peruvian and broader South American- Spanish-speaking populations.

Strengths and Limitations: Spanish versions of the ACE-R and ACE-III demonstrate strong psychometric properties, practical administration time, and utility for differentiating dementia subtypes. However, validation studies remain limited to Spain, Argentina, Chile, and Peru, with notable gaps in Mexico and other Latin American countries. Given the significant effects of age and education, careful consideration of normative applicability across diverse Spanish-speaking populations is essential.

Mini-Cog

The Mini-Cog is a rapid screening tool combining three-word recall and clock drawing to assess memory, executive, and visuospatial functions, typically administered in under three minutes (Borson et al, 2000).

Validation of the Mini-Cog in Spanish-speaking populations shows mixed results. In primary care (Carnero-Pardo et al, 2013), including a sample of 131 older healthy adults and 176 with mild cognitive impairment, the Mini-Cog showed moderate diagnostic accuracy (AUC = 0.78) of impaired individuals; this diagnostic accuracy was lower than the MMSE and the Clock Drawing Test, with best performance at a one-half cut-off (sensitivity = 0.60, specificity = 0.90). In a neurology clinic (Carnero-Pardo et al, 2022) including 581 older adults, diagnostic accuracy was higher (AUC = 0.88) with a two-thirds cut-off (sensitivity = 0.90, specificity = 0.71), though instruments demonstrated reduced diagnostic utility among low-education groups, where the AUC dropped to 0.74 ± 0.05.

Strengths and Limitations: The Spanish Mini-Cog is quick, practical, and useful for initial screening, especially in time-limited settings. However, its accuracy varies by education level and clinical context, underscoring the need for follow-up with more comprehensive assessments when impairment is suspected.

Six-Item Screener

The Six-Item Screener (SIS) is a brief cognitive assessment derived from the MMSE, consisting of three orientation items and a three-word recall (Callahan et al, 2002). It can be administered in 2–3 minutes, in person or by phone, making it useful for large studies and time-limited clinical settings.

The SIS is a core part of the cognitive battery in the Hispanic Community Health Study/Study of Latinos (HCHS/SOL) and SOL-INCA, alongside the Brief Spanish English Verbal Learning Test (B-SEVLT), Word Fluency, and Digit Symbol Substitution tests.

The original validation of the SIS (Callahan et al, 2002) showed good psychometric properties, with a cut-off of ≤3, yielding 88.7% sensitivity and 88.0% specificity for dementia, comparable to the MMSE (cut-off ≤23; sensitivity 95.2%, and specificity 86.7%). In the SOL-INCA study (N = 9,309), a cut-off of ≤4 defined low cognitive status, classifying about 10% of Hispanic/Latino participants as impaired (Breton et al, 2021; Vasquez et al, 2022). However, measurement equivalence analyses revealed that one SIS item was more difficult in Spanish, suggesting language-based bias that may affect cross-group comparisons (Goodman et al, 2021). Within SOL-INCA, the SIS has been widely applied to examine cognitive aging and risk factors such as cardiovascular health and cognitive stimulation in diverse Hispanic/Latino populations (Vasquez et al, 2022; Gonzalez et al, 2020).

Strengths and Limitations: The SIS is brief, practical, and psychometrically sound, with demonstrated value in research on Hispanic/Latino cognitive aging. Yet, language-based biases and limited domain coverage mean it should be used as a screening tool rather than as a standalone diagnostic measure.

GLOBAL COGNITIVE SCREENING MEASURES/NEUROPSYCHOLOGICAL BATTERIES

Consortium to Establish a Registry for Alzheimer's Disease

The Consortium to Establish a Registry for Alzheimer's Disease (CERAD) battery (Morris et al, 1988) includes seven subtests, the MMSE, semantic fluency (animals), word list learning, word list recall, word list recognition, 15-item Boston Naming Test (BNT-15), constructional praxis, and has several Spanish-language norms.

Aguirre-Acevedo et al. (2007) adapted the CERAD Neuropsychological Battery for Spanish speakers in Antioquia, Colombia (CERAD-Col) and assessed its reliability and validity in 848 controls and 151 AD patients aged >50. Controls were recruited from senior groups in the Aburrá Valley, while AD cases included 90 retrospective medical records and 61 new diagnoses from the *Grupo de Neurociencias de Antioquia* (1994–2004). Means and SDs were reported; internal consistency (Cronbach's α) and test-retest reliability (intraclass correlation coefficient) were established. Construct validity was supported through factor analysis, correlations with functional scales, and group comparisons (controls versus AD).

Henao-Arboleda et al. (2010) expanded earlier work by Aguirre-Acevedo et al. (2007) to further validate neuropsychological measures for diagnosing AD in Colombians over age 50. Validity assessments included content, face, construct, and criterion validity, along with internal consistency. Performances were compared across 848 controls, 36 individuals with MCI, and 151 with AD. Cut-off points were provided by age, education, and gender. Analyses included descriptive statistics, Cronbach's α, ICC, and Mann-Whitney U tests for group comparisons. The authors concluded that the battery is suitable for evaluating neurodegenerative conditions in Colombian populations and those with similar sociodemographic profiles.

Torres et al. (2021) provided Colombian norms using 2,673 cognitively unimpaired adults (ages 18–86; M = 32.94, SD = 12.10) from the Antioquia region. Education ranged 1–25 years (M = 8.89, SD = 4.34), with stratification by age and education. In addition to the CERAD subtests, nine measures were added:

- Memory Impairment Screening (MIS) (Buschke et al, 1999), adapted to Spanish by Romero-Vanegas et al. (2010)
- Memory Capacity Test (MCT) (Buschke, 1984), adapted to Spanish by Romero-Vanegas et al. (2010)
- Rey-Osterrieth Complex Figure (RCFT) (Osterrieth, 1944b)
- Raven's Progressive Matrices, Part A (Raven, 1938)
- Trail Making Test-A (TMT-A) (Reitan and Wolfson, 1985a)
- Weschler Adult Intelligence Scale, Third Edition, Digit Symbol (WAIS-III) (Wechsler, 1997)
- "A" Cancellation Test (Ardila, Rosselli, and Puente, 1994)
- Phonemic Fluency (FAS) (Benton and Hamsher, 1976)
- Wisconsin Card Sorting Test (WCST-48) (Nelson, 1976)

Analyses examined associations with age and education: education correlated with semantic fluency, BNT-15, word list learning, Raven's Progressive Matrices, and Digit Symbol; age was negatively associated with visuoconstruction, delayed recall, Digit Symbol, and phonemic fluency, but positively correlated with TMT-A.

Fillenbaum et al. (2007) translated the CERAD Battery into Spanish using forward-backward translation and established norms stratified by disease severity (CDR 0–3). The sample included 88 non-demented controls and 140 AD patients from the University of Southern California, plus 102 Spanish-speaking dementia patients from the University of Pennsylvania. Controls outperformed mild AD patients, and performance declined with disease severity. Analyses included descriptive statistics, logistic regression for age and gender effects, and sensitivity/specificity estimates distinguishing controls (CDR 0) from mild AD (CDR 1).

Carrión-Baralt et al. (2009) examined the CERAD Word List and other neuropsychological data in 81 Spanish-speaking nondemented nonagenarians from Puerto Rico and 62 from the New York area, comparing demographic effects and cross-cultural performance. Education emerged as the strongest predictor: when controlled, Puerto Rican nonagenarians performed comparably to white, English-speaking peers in New York. The Puerto Rico sample (M age = 92.82, SD = 2.27; M education = 8.87, SD = 5.21; 57.3% female) was recruited from senior centers, living facilities, agencies, and the community.

The New York sample (M age = 92.75, SD = 2.52; M education = 15.76, SD = 3.10; 64.5% female) came from VA- and university-based recruitment, community talks, and ads. All participants were nondemented (CDR = 0). Analyses included descriptive statistics, regression for age, education, and sex, and ANCOVA for between-sample comparisons.

Sosa et al. (2009) provided normative data for four components of the 10/66 Dementia Research Group battery, including the CERAD Word List, stratified by age, sex, and education. The study included participants without dementia from Cuba, the Dominican Republic, Venezuela, Peru, Mexico, China, and India. Means and SDs were reported by site and demographic group. General linear models assessed the effects of age, sex, and education across sites, as well as site-level differences by region (Latin America versus China/India) and by rural–urban status.

Guerrero-Berroa et al. (2016) provided age- and sex-stratified norms and examined demographic effects on neuropsychological performance in Spanish-speaking nonagenarians with low education. The study included 95 cognitively normal elderly from Costa Rica (M age = 93.7, SD = 3.4; M education = 2.9 years, range 0–6; 68.3% female), 15 of whom had no formal education. A comparison group of 23 Puerto Rican participants (ages 90–99, <7 years of education, CDR = 0) was also included. Regression analyses assessed the impact of age, sex, and education; ANOVAs tested performance differences by age, sex, and education categories; ANCOVA compared Costa Rican and Puerto Rican groups, controlling for demographics.

O'Bryant et al. (2018) developed age- and education-stratified norms for a comprehensive neuropsychological battery in 797 Mexican Americans aged 40+ from Texas. Measures included the MMSE, AMNART, WMS-III (Logical Memory I/II; Visual Reproduction I/II; Digit Span), CERAD, Rey Auditory Verbal Learning Test (RAVLT), Executive Interview (25-item version—EXIT25), Clock Drawing Executive Test, Parts 1 and 2 (CLOX 1 & 2), Trail Making Test A & B, Boston Naming Test (BNT), Controlled Oral Word Association (COWA), and Animal Naming. All participants had a CDR global score of 0 and consensus-confirmed normal cognition. Norms were based on participants' preferred language of test administration (English or Spanish) and included both urban and rural residents.

Zuno-Reyes et al. (2023) developed regression-based continuous norms for the Mexican adaptation of the CERAD using both linear regression (LR) and nonlinear quantile regression (NQR), with age, sex, and education as covariates. The sample included 392 native Spanish-speaking Mexican adults aged 18–59 (M = 38.8, SD = 11.8; M education = 10.4 years, SD = 5.1; 50.3% women) recruited from municipalities in Jalisco. Analyses proceeded in three stages: 1) calculation of raw percentiles, 2) regression-based norms using age, sex, and education, and 3) NQR-based norms excluding age and sex effects following Abbott et al. (2019). The authors concluded that NQR provided greater accuracy than LR for characterizing cognitive performance.

Strengths and Limitations: The CERAD neuropsychological battery demonstrates several notable strengths and limitations across its adaptations and validations in Spanish-speaking populations. Strengths include its extensive validation history, large and diverse normative samples, and inclusion of reliability and validity indices in multiple studies, ensuring robust psychometric support. Adaptations such as the CERAD-Col have provided culturally and linguistically relevant versions with stratified norms by age, education, and gender, enhancing diagnostic accuracy in older adults and individuals with varying educational backgrounds. Expanded versions, like those by Torres et al. (2021) and O'Bryant et al. (2018) further strengthened the battery's applicability by including additional measures, bilingual testing, and broader demographic representation. However, limitations persist, including uneven stratification across studies, small subgroup sizes, and restricted generalizability to non-Colombian or bilingual populations. Some studies relied on convenience sampling or lacked full psychometric analyses, such as test–retest reliability or construct validity, while others provided translations without complete cultural adaptation. Overall, the CERAD battery remains a valuable and versatile tool for assessing cognitive function across Spanish-speaking groups, though future work should aim to improve demographic balance, bilingual validation, and cultural specificity.

Batería Neuropsicológica en Español

Batería Neuropsicológica en Español is a brief neuropsychological tool comprising eight tests evaluating cognitive performance, including attention, executive functions, learning, and memory (Artiola et al, 1999).

The sample comprises Spanish-speaking adults from Madrid, Spain, and the U.S./Mexico border. The sample comprised 390 cognitively intact adults, 205 residing in Madrid, Spain, and 185 from the U.S./Mexico border. The sample ranged from 18 to ≥ 65 years of age, with education ranging from 0 to ≥ 16 years. Stepwise regression analysis was conducted to evaluate the impact of demographic variables. As such, normative data were stratified by age, education, and country of origin.

Strengths and Limitations: A key strength of this battery lies in the normative data, which are stratified by age, education, and country of origin, enhancing its cross-cultural relevance and applicability across diverse Spanish-speaking adults. Limitations include its relatively narrow age range (18–≥65), which may reduce its utility in older adult populations, particularly important in aging and dementia research.

NEUROPSI Atención y Memoria (NEUROPSI Attention and Memory)

Ostrosky-Solís et al. (2007) developed the NEUROPSI Attention and Memory, a neuropsychological battery assessing orientation, attention/concentration, executive functions, working memory, and immediate and delayed verbal/visual memory.

Norms were based on 521 cognitively intact community volunteers from urban and rural regions of Mexico (Mexico City, Colima, Guadalajara, and Zacatecas) collected over four years. Participants ranged from 6–85 years (education 0–22 years). Age groups were stratified into nine categories (6–7, 8–9, 10–11, 12–13, 14–15, 16–30, 31–55, 56–64, and 65–85), and education into three levels (0–3, 4–9, and 10–22 years). Factor analysis identified six factors accounting for about 63% of the variance:

- Attentional-executive (.62–70)
- Contextual-executive memory (.45–79)
- Verbal memory (.70–81)
- Selective/sustained attention and orientation (.40–70)
- Attentional working memory (.47–69)
- Place/person orientation (.88–89)

Age effects were examined via one-way ANOVA; education effects were examined via MANOVA.

Strengths and Limitations: Strengths include a wide age range and stratification by education, enhancing sensitivity to cognitive changes (e.g., early-onset AD). Limitations include a lack of reported psychometric indices (validity, reliability, sensitivity, specificity), generalizability restricted to Mexican populations, and a ceiling effect at 85 years of age.

Dementia Rating Scale

The Spanish Translation Dementia Rating Scale-Second edition (ST-DRS-2) (Strutt et al, 2012) is a global screening measure for those with suspected neurodegenerative diseases, adapted from the Mattis Dementia Rating Scale-2 (MDRS-2) (Jurica, Leitten, and Mattis, 2001). It includes five scales: attention, initiation/perseveration, construction, conceptualization, and memory. The translation and back-translation process was straightforward, given the MDRS-2's simple design.

The normative sample included 157 Spanish-speaking cognitively intact adults (ages 50–80; 61.8% women; 6–19 years of education) from 15 Latin American countries, all residing in the U.S. and with low-moderate acculturation. Additional groups included 60 Spanish-speaking dementia patients (Houston, Texas, and Puerto Rico) and 30 non-Hispanic, English-speaking controls. Linguistic status was evaluated using the Expressive Vocabulary Test and the Marin Acculturation Scale. Norms were stratified by age and education. Sensitivity/specificity analyses indicated that a total score <125 yielded 96% sensitivity and 50% specificity, while a memory score <17 yielded 99% sensitivity and 72% specificity.

Strengths and Limitations: Strengths include a brief, targeted global measure with a diverse Spanish-speaking sample across multiple countries. Limitations include potential construct validity issues in lower-acculturated individuals, over-adjustment for higher education, modest sample size, exclusion of participants with <6 years of education, monolingual-only norms, and lack of broader psychometric indices.

Neuropsychological Screening Battery for Hispanics

Neuropsychological Screening Battery for Hispanics (NeSBHIS) is a comprehensive screening battery adapted from the World Health Organization (WHO) battery, assessing language, memory, visuospatial functioning, mental control, reasoning, and psychomotor abilities. Administration takes about 80 minutes (Ponton et al, 1996).

Based on 342 cognitively intact adults from Los Angeles, including Spanish-speaking monolinguals (70%) and bilinguals. Most were of Mexican origin (62%), with additional representation from Central America (15%) and other countries (25%). Participants ranged from 16–75 years of age (M = 38.4, SD = 13.5), divided into four age groups (16–29, 30–39, 40–49, and 50–75). Education ranged from 1–20 years (M = 10.7, SD = 5.1), categorized as <10 years (n = 129) or ≥10 years (n = 171). Normative data were stratified by age, education, and gender in a 4 × 2 × 2 model.

Strengths and Limitations: Strengths include focus on U.S.-residing Spanish speakers and bilinguals, making norms clinically relevant for Hispanic populations in the U.S. Limitations are the relatively small sample, limited stratification for older adults, and outdated norms (collected almost 30 years ago).

The National Institute of Health Toolbox Cognition Battery

The National Institute of Health Toolbox Cognition Battery (NIHTB-CB) (Weintraub et al, 2014; Gershon et al, 2020; Casaletto et al, 2016) is a brief computerized battery available in English and Spanish, taking about 30 minutes to administer. It includes seven subtests covering six domains (attention, executive functioning, memory, processing speed, working memory, and language) and yields three composite scores: fluid, crystallized, and total cognition. The fluid composite consists of five tasks (dimensional change card sort, flanker, picture sequence memory, list sorting, and pattern comparison), while the crystallized composite includes picture vocabulary and oral reading recognition. The total composite reflects the average of the two.

The sample included 408 neurologically healthy, Spanish-speaking adults (ages 18–85; M = 44.1, SD = 16.7; M education = 10.7 years, SD = 4.3; 35% male) recruited across 10 U.S. sites (Atlanta, Georgia; Chicago–Oak Brook, Illinois; Cincinnati, Ohio; Columbus, Ohio; Dallas, Texas; Los Angeles, California; Minneapolis, Minnesota; Philadelphia, Pennsylvania; Phoenix, Arizona; and St. Louis; Missouri). Norms provide uncorrected, age-corrected, and demographically corrected scores (age, gender, and education). Spanish and English norms are distinct, and participants may select their preferred testing language.

Strengths and Limitations: Strengths include brevity, computerized administration, and broad domain coverage. Limitations include reliance on self-selected language preference, lack of cultural/acculturation or immigration data, and uncertain generalizability across diverse Spanish-speaking populations.

Repeatable Battery for the Assessment of Neuropsychological Status—Form A

Repeatable Battery for the Assessment of Neuropsychological Status (RBANS) (Randolph et al, 1998) is a screening tool with 12 subtests measuring attention, visuospatial/constructional skills, language, and immediate and delayed memory. Attention is assessed with digit span and coding; visuospatial/construction with figure copy and line orientation; language with picture naming and semantic fluency; immediate memory with list learning and story memory; and delayed memory with list recall, list recognition, story recall, and figure recall.

Encinas et al. (2012) translated and adapted the RBANS to Spanish and tested it in 73 participants from Spain: 25 males with a mean age of 54 years and 9.72 years of education, and 48 females with a mean age of 53 years and 10.29 years of education. The battery was translated using the translation-back-translation method (with slight differences). An overall reliability coefficient with a Cronbach alpha of 0.73 was obtained in the translation and adaptation of the RBANS. De La Torre et al. (2014) tested the RBANS reliability and sensitivity and obtained normative data of a Spanish adaptation of the RBANS. In this study, 50 participants with AD and 336 healthy participants stratified according to the Spanish Census, with different levels of education, were tested with the RBANS (Form A). More recently, Muntal et al. (2020) provided normative data from the RBANS-E (Spanish-language version of RBANS form A) for a Spanish population aged 20–89 years with diverse levels of education. The study included 609 subjects who were evaluated at baseline with a short interview, a cognitive screening test (Mini-Mental State Examination), and a functional scale (Rapid Disability Rating Scale) in addition to the RBANS-E.

In the U.S., Hall et al. (2018) obtained norms for the RBANS in a sample of 136 cognitively intact Mexican American adults (ages not specified) from the FRONTIER project. Participants were tested in their preferred language (67 Spanish, 69 English). Education ranged from 0–18 years (M = 8.2, SD = 4.0). Performance was predicted by stepwise regression with age, education, gender, and language in the model. Normative tables were created for English and Spanish-speaking Mexican Americans. Generated RBANS normative references are provided for unadjusted raw scores as well as output adjusted by education level.

Strengths and Limitations: The RBANS shows solid reliability and validity in its Spanish adaptations, with rigorous translation procedures and large normative samples spanning diverse ages and education levels. Studies in Spain and among Mexican Americans have enhanced its clinical utility and cultural relevance. However, limitations include small sample sizes in some studies, limited cross-cultural generalizability beyond these populations, and incomplete psychometric data. Differences in educational systems, regional dialects, and cultural contexts may further affect interpretation, highlighting the need for continued adaptation and validation across diverse Spanish-speaking populations.

Spanish and English Neuropsychological Assessment Scales

Spanish and English Neuropsychological Assessment Scales (SENAS) is a brief neuropsychological battery of 13 tasks assessing conceptual thinking, semantic memory, attention span, episodic memory, nonverbal–spatial skills, and verbal abilities. Subtests include verbal and non-verbal conceptual thinking, object naming, picture association, verbal and visual attention span, word list learning I/II, spatial configuration learning, pattern recognition, spatial localization, verbal comprehension, and verbal expression (Mungas et al, 2004).

Norms were developed from 1,374 cognitively intact U.S.-residing older adults (ages 60–101; education 0–19 years), divided into three groups: English-speaking white (n = 341), English-speaking Hispanics (n = 357), and Spanish-speaking Hispanics (n = 676). Mean education was 14.1 years for whites, 11.0 years for English-speaking Hispanics, and 4.6 years for Spanish-speaking Hispanics. Average ages were 72.9, 70.3, and 71.0 years, respectively. Item response theory (IRT) and covariance structure analysis (CSA) were used to refine scales. Internal consistency ranged from .73 to .92 across groups, with mean reliabilities of .85 to .88. English and Spanish versions demonstrated good comparability, though only moderate interscale correlations.

Strengths and Limitations: Strengths include robust psychometric properties, minimal floor/ceiling effects, and strong cross-language matching between English and Spanish versions. Limitations include a lack of executive functioning measures and the need for further construct validation.

Neuropsychological Assessment of the Spanish Speaker

Ardila et al. (1994) published the Neuropsychological Assessment of the Spanish Speaker, a compilation of widely used tests translated into Spanish with accompanying psychometric data and normative references. Cognitive domains include attention/orientation, language, memory, and visuospatial/praxis abilities. Thirteen tests are covered, with materials provided in the appendix of Ardila's book.

Several normative samples were used. One sample of 180 participants was divided into three education levels and three age groups (10 participants per cell). Another included 360 participants divided into three education levels and five age ranges. A third sample of 200 participants used two education levels (illiterate versus professional) and five age ranges. For the Wechsler Memory Scale, 300 participants were stratified by five age groups and three education levels. Norms are provided for nine tests: A Cancellation, Digit Symbol, Spanish Naming, Verbal Fluency, Verbal Serial Learning Curve, Digit Span, Memory for Unfamiliar Faces, Rey–Osterrieth Complex Figure, and Finger-Tapping.

Strengths and Limitations: Strengths include providing Spanish translations of common English-language measures, facilitating comparability across populations, and offering some normative data. Limitations include outdated norms, small subgroup sizes, and simplified stratification schemes (binary or limited education/age categories), which reduce representativeness.

Rowland Universal Dementia Assessment Scale

Rowland Universal Dementia Assessment Scale (RUDAS) is a brief multicultural cognitive screener designed for individuals with lower educational attainment (Storey et al, 2004). It consists of six items assessing memory, praxis, language, judgment, drawing, and body orientation, with a total score out of 30.

Coelho-Guimarães et al. (2021) validated the RUDAS in rural, semi-rural, and urban areas of Spain with 150 older adults (61 men, 89 women; M age = 76.3, SD = 7.1). Participants were divided into five age bands (65–69, 70–74, 75–79, 80–84, and 85+). Most came from rural settings (n = 100), with fewer from semi-rural (n = 46) and urban (n = 8) areas. Education was categorized qualitatively: illiterate (5%), elementary (58%), secondary/"instituto" (29%), high school (7%), and university (1%). CDR scores classified participants as cognitively intact (75%), MCI (13%), mild dementia (10%), or moderate dementia (1%). Test-retest reliability (10-day interval, n = 71) was strong (Spearman = .665; Pearson r = .712), as was inter-rater reliability (n = 46, Cronbach's α = .876). Discriminant validity showed good sensitivity and specificity distinguishing controls, MCI, and dementia, with especially strong accuracy for differentiating MCI from dementia (sensitivity = .900, specificity = .941).

Strengths and Limitations: Strengths include the inclusion of diverse regions within Spain and robust psychometric data (e.g., reliability, PPV/NPV, and sensitivity/specificity). Limitations include restricted generalizability outside Spain and potential cultural/educational influences unique to that context.

INTELLECTUAL FUNCTIONING

Wechsler Adult Intelligence Scale-III

The Wechsler Adult Intelligence Scale-III (WAIS-III)—Spain (Wechsler, 2001) is the Spanish adaptation of the WAIS-III, standardized on 1,369 Spaniards aged 15–94 years (49% men, 51% women), primarily from urban areas and stratified across four education levels. The scale includes 14 subtests divided into verbal IQ (VIQ) and the manipulative scale (MIQ). VIQ incorporates the Verbal Comprehension Index (VCI) and Working Memory Index (WMI), with tasks such as vocabulary, similarities, information, arithmetic, digit span, and letter-number sequencing, as well as a comprehension subtest outside the indexes. The MIQ encompasses the Perceptual Organization Index (POI) and the Processing Speed Index (PSI), which include block design, matrix reasoning, incomplete figures, digit symbol-coding, and symbol search, along with additional tasks like puzzles and picture arrangement.

Cross-national comparisons by Funes et al. (2016) revealed systematic differences when Spanish norms were compared with those from Mexico, Puerto Rico, and the U.S. On digit span, Spaniards consistently scored lower than U.S. peers across all ages, while results on digit symbol-coding were equivalent in younger adults (16–34) but lower for Spaniards over age 35. Block design showed the reverse: younger Spaniards outperformed U.S. peers, but older Spaniards scored lower. Comparisons with the Mexican sample revealed further variability, with younger Mexicans (25–34) performing below Spaniards on digit span, but older Mexicans (55–69 and 70+) outperforming Spaniards on digit span and block design.

Reliability estimates for the WAIS-III-S were high (IQ and Index scores = 0.87–0.97; subtests = 0.77–0.98), comparable to U.S. norms and stronger than the Mexican version (0.70–0.87). Validity studies, including work by Renteria et al. (2008) generally support the test's utility, though letter-number sequencing demonstrated weaker consistency. Some evidence suggests the Spanish WAIS-III may underestimate ability compared to external criteria, indicating possible test bias in certain groups.

Strengths and Limitations: The WAIS-III-S is a psychometrically solid measure, with high reliability and good validity for all subtests except Letter Number Sequencing. Interpretation requires attention to cultural and demographic differences. Spanish and Mexican norms appear particularly problematic for adults over 70, as the former may underestimate and the latter may overestimate cognitive deficits. These discrepancies, likely shaped by educational, socioeconomic, and health factors, underscore the importance of careful selection of normative data and awareness of potential subtest- and age-specific biases.

WAIS-III—Mexico

The WAIS-III—Mexico underwent several stages of development. A preliminary version of the norms appeared in 2001, followed by expanded age-based norms in 2003 and a 2004 revision that attempted to statistically correct for the underestimation of IQ. However, serious concerns have been raised about the validity of these norms. Suen and Greenspan (2009) argued that, whether based on the Hispanic American version (1999), the preliminary Mexican version (2001), or the 2003 update, the test lacked reliability, had no meaningful normative reference population, excluded certain groups, and used an inappropriate confidence interval method for interpreting low scores in legal and clinical contexts. These limitations led some authors to suggest withdrawing the Mexican norms altogether.

The normative sample included about 1,000 participants from four regions of Mexico (center, north, west, and southeast), drawn from urban areas and stratified by education level. While age and regional distribution were relatively balanced, the sample contained a disproportionate number of individuals with higher levels of education, making it less representative of the general population.

Strengths and Limitations: Some strengths were noted, such as acceptable reliability in certain age groups and reasonable sensitivity and specificity for detecting neurological disorders (e.g., Alzheimer's, Huntington's, and Parkinson's). Key problems included a lack of clarity on sample characteristics, an absence of census-based representation, and no true normalization of scores. Instead, the manual relied on linear transformations of raw scores using anchor points, making percentile interpretations questionable. Escobedo and Hollingworth (2009) further highlighted the absence of reported reliability data in the manual, with most coefficients falling only within "acceptable" ranges and no reliability information for the latest version. Importantly, older adults and individuals with intellectual disabilities were underrepresented, further limiting the generalizability of the norms.

Escala de Inteligencia Wechsler para Adultos-III—Puerto Rico

The Escala de Inteligencia Wechsler para Adultos-III (EIWA-III)—Puerto Rico (Wechsler, 2008) is the Puerto Rican adaptation of the WAIS-III, developed with the Ponce School of Medicine to ensure cultural validity. It includes the full range of WAIS-III subtests, assessing key processes such as the Verbal Comprehension Index (VCI), Working Memory Index (WMI), Perceptual Organization Index (POI), and Processing Speed Index (PSI), grouped under Verbal IQ (VIQ) and Performance IQ (PIQ). It was normed on individuals ages 16–64, and it requires approximately 60–95 minutes to complete.

Standardization was conducted with 330 Puerto Rican adults (52% men, 48% women), stratified across five education levels (0–8, 9–11, 12, 13–15, and >16 years). Psychometric studies indicate high reliability and validity, with strong internal consistency, temporal stability, and effect sizes 0.04–0.48, confirming robustness across subtests (Pons et al, 2008). Its four-factor structure mirrors the original WAIS-III, supporting content, concurrent, predictive, and discriminant validity.

> **Strengths and Limitations:** The EIWA-III-PR provides a culturally adapted, psychometrically sound tool for assessing intellectual functioning in Puerto Rican adults. However, its relatively small normative sample (n = 330) and limited age range (up to 64 years) restrict generalization, highlighting the need for expanded norms in older adults.

Wechsler Adult Intelligence Scale-IV (WAIS-IV)

WAIS-IV—Chile

A total of 887 participants (ages 16–90) were initially recruited and classified by education: low (<8 years), medium (9–15 years), and high (>17 years, university/postgraduate). Parental education was also recorded for those with 15–25 years of schooling. Because only 12 of 15 subtests were administered to participants over 70, the final sample included 672 individuals (M age = 36.9, SD = 17.1; 50.5% women) from seven regions of Chile (Metropolitan Region, Bíobío, Arica y Parinacota, Tarapacá, Antofagasta, Araucanía, and Magallanes). Education and gender were evenly distributed, except at age 75, where women predominated (Duggan et al, 2019; Rosas et al, 2014).

Psychometric evaluation showed strong reliability and validity. Internal consistency was high (Cronbach's $\alpha = 0.941$ overall; 0.628–0.937 across subtests). Test-retest reliability was assumed from the original WAIS-IV. Validity analyses, including confirmatory factor analysis and correlation matrices, supported the expected factor structure, with stronger correlations among subtests within the same index (e.g., vocabulary–comprehension $r = 0.72$; arithmetic-digit span $r = 0.63$). Logistic regression and Mantel-Haenszel tests identified no regional differences, modest gender effects (men outperforming women), and clear education effects, with higher education linked to higher scores. Bias analyses showed minimal item bias, limited to age in one subtest.

WAIS-IV—Colombia, Mexico, Spain

Four comprised scores corresponded to differing factorial indices, verbal comprehension (similarities, vocabulary, information) with supplementary tests of comprehension (VCI), perceptual reasoning (PRI; block design, matrix reasoning, picture completion) with supplementary subtests of balances and incomplete figures, working memory (WMI; digit span, arithmetic) with supplementary subtests such as letter-number sequencing, and processing speed (PSI; digit symbol-coding, symbol search) with subtests of cancellation, as well as general ability. The WAIS-IV scores included the indices (VCI, PRI, WMI, and PSI) and the FSIQ.

According to Duggan et al. (2019), who examined WAIS-IV normative data from Colombia, Chile, Mexico, Spain, Canada, and the U.S., the Mexican norms were based on 1,450 Spanish-speaking participants aged 16–90, divided into 13 age groups. However, little information on educational background was provided. In contrast, the Colombian WAIS-IV was standardized with 156 participants stratified by age, sex, geographic region, and socioeconomic-education variables. For Colombian executives (n = 305), WAIS-IV scores (FSIQ and subtest indices: VCI, PRI, WMI, PSI) were recalculated using norms from six countries, yielding multiple score sets per individual. Thirteen age groups were defined in both Colombia and Mexico based on census data (16–90 years). In Colombia and Chile, education was not measured directly but inferred from socioeconomic strata: low (≤8 years), medium (9–17 years), and high (≥17 years), with an even distribution across groups (33% each). Converted to ISCED units, 67% of Colombians fell into levels 0–3 (high school or less), similar to Chile, while 83% of Mexicans fell in this category and only 16% in levels 4–8 (postsecondary).

Results indicated strong similarity between Colombian and Chilean norms, with scores within one-third SD for FSIQ and index measures. Mexican norms showed higher concordance with Colombian norms for FSIQ (82%) and VCI (78%) but lower agreement for PRI (31%), WMI (21%), and PSI (17%). Classification agreement between Mexico and Colombia ranged from 66% for FSIQ to 32% for PSI, typically differing by one or two categories, though VCI was occasionally higher. Subtest-level agreement was also high between Colombia and Chile (100%), whereas Mexico showed more variability, with concordance ranging from 84% (cancellation) to 100% (vocabulary).

The WAIS-IV Spain underwent substantial modifications, including item substitutions, score adjustments, and removal of some tasks for time efficiency. It is administered to individuals aged 16–89, though certain tasks (e.g., balances, letters and numbers, cancellations) are limited to ages 16–69. Validity analyses showed medium correlations overall, with stronger correlations for tasks measuring the same constructs (0.50–0.63) than for different ones (0.12–0.64). The scale also showed high correlations with WAIS-III tasks (0.67–0.86) and indices (0.80–0.92). Reliability was strong, with Cronbach's alpha ranging from 0.72–0.93 for subtests and 0.87–0.97 for indices, and test-retest correlations from 0.66–0.88 at the subtest level and 0.81–0.94 for indices.

Strengths and Limitations: The WAIS-IV is a well-established measure that captures multiple cognitive domains (VCI, PRI, WMI, PSI, and FSIQ) and demonstrates strong reliability and validity across contexts. Notably, Colombian and Chilean norms are highly consistent, and the Spanish adaptation shows solid psychometric performance, including robust test-retest reliability and construct validity. At the same time, important limitations remain; normative samples differ in size and representativeness, with Mexican norms providing limited educational stratification and showing weaker concordance with Colombian norms for several indices. Moreover, modifications in the Spanish version and the use of socioeconomic status as a proxy for education in some countries reduce comparability and may constrain the cross-cultural generalizability of findings.

Reynolds Intellectual Assessment Scales

The Reynolds Intellectual Assessment Scales (RIAS) include four core subtests yielding a Composite Intelligence Index (CIX), derived from the Verbal Intelligence Index (VIX; guess what, verbal reasoning) and the Nonverbal Intelligence Index (NIX; odd-item out, what's missing). A Composite Memory Index (CMX) is also provided from verbal memory (recall of sentences/stories) and nonverbal memory (recall/recognition of visual images). Together, the six subtests can be used to estimate general intelligence ("g") (Reynolds and Kamphaus, 2013).

Norms were established on a U.S. sample of 2,438 individuals aged 3–94, stratified by age, gender, ethnicity, education, and geography, and broadly representative of census distributions (White 61–70%, African American 7.6–15%, and Hispanic 4.8–18%). Standardization occurred between 1999–2002 across 41 states. Factor analyses supported a two-factor solution (verbal and nonverbal domains) across demographic groups. The Spanish version is published as RÍAS, *Escalas de Inteligencia de Reynolds*.

Psychometrics are strong: internal consistency and test-retest reliability were high (α = .90–95 for subtests; .94–96 for indexes; stability coefficients .83–91), and interscorer reliability approached 1.00. Validity was supported through theory-driven factor analysis and correlations with Wechsler scales and academic achievement.

Strengths and Limitations: RIAS is efficient and adaptable for school and clinical use, offering a co-normed working memory component while reducing administration time without loss of rigor. Limitations include reliance on motor and visual-motor speed, as well as some sensitivity to reading ability and potential differential item functioning by gender and ethnicity.

Batería III

The Batería III (Muñoz-Sandoval et al, 2005) is the parallel Spanish version of the Woodcock-Johnson III Test of Cognitive Abilities (Woodcock-Johnson, 2007), grounded in Cattel-Horn-Carroll (CHC) theory (McGrew et al, 2023). It includes the COG battery (31 tests) assessing general intelligence, broad and narrow cognitive abilities, memory, processing speed, and executive functions, and the APROV battery (22 tests) measuring oral language, reading, mathematics, writing, phonological awareness, and academic knowledge. All materials are in Spanish, designed for ages 2–90+, with each subtest taking about 5–10 minutes to complete. When paired with the WJ IV, it allows direct Spanish-English skill comparisons.

It was standardized on a large, diverse U.S. sample (ages 2–90+), with age- and grade-based norms, the Batería III demonstrates strong reliability (most coefficients ≥ .90) and validity for educational, clinical, and research use.

Strengths and Limitations: The Batería III Woodcock-Muñoz offers a comprehensive, reliable, and culturally appropriate assessment of cognitive and academic abilities for Spanish-speaking populations, with strong psychometric properties and computerized scoring that enhances accuracy and efficiency. Its design reduces the risk of misdiagnosis by providing norms tailored for Spanish speakers and allows direct comparison with English versions, making it highly versatile across educational, clinical, and research settings. However, limitations include variability in cultural and linguistic relevance across different Spanish-speaking regions, potential influences of bilingualism or dialect differences on performance, and possible gaps in normative sample representativeness, which may restrict generalizability for some subgroups. Moreover, interpretation may not always fully capture the cultural and educational backgrounds of examinees, leading to potential under- or overestimation of abilities.

Batería IV

The Batería IV (LaForte et al, 2019) Woodcock-Muñoz is the Spanish adaptation of the WJ IV, published in 2019, and provides parallel forms of the most educationally and diagnostically useful WJ IV tests. Grounded in Cattell-Horn-Carroll (CHC) theory, it offers two main batteries: the Test of Cognitive Abilities (COG; Tests 1–7) and the Test of Achievement (APROV; Tests 1–6), with clusters that assess broad cognitive abilities and academic skills. When combined with the WJ IV Tests of Oral Language, it enables a comprehensive evaluation of cognitive, achievement, and oral language abilities across English and Spanish. Both versions rely on the same normative framework, derived from a nationally representative U.S. sample of 7,416 individuals spanning ages 2–90+, with stratification across children, K–12 students, college students, and adults.

Strengths and Limitations: Batería IV provides a reliable, valid, and culturally appropriate assessment for Spanish speakers, developed in line with the Standards for Educational and Psychological Testing (American Educational Research Association, 2014). Its strengths include rigorous validation, online scoring that reduces errors, and the use of a CHC-based framework consistent with WJ IV, ensuring interpretive comparability. Limitations remain in cultural generalizability, as regional variations in the Spanish language and educational systems may affect test interpretation for subgroups not fully represented in the U.S.-based norming sample.

PREMORBID LITERACY

Literacy substantially influences neuropsychological test performance, as many standardized cognitive assessments draw upon skills that are directly or indirectly shaped by reading and writing proficiency. More broadly, literacy serves as a proxy not only for exposure to formal education and structured learning environments, but also the quality of formal as well as informal education (Manly et al, 2002). All of these experiences contribute to the development of higher-order cognitive processes, particularly those assessed by measures of language, processing speed, and executive function. When literacy is not adequately considered (in addition to years of education), clinicians risk misattributing low test scores (e.g., to neuropathology) rather than to differences in the quality of educational experience, leading to potential diagnostic inaccuracies in populations that may have limited formal schooling.

Word Accentuation Test (Chicago, Spain, Argentina, New York, TMAANS)

The Word Accentuation Test (WAT) (Del Ser et al, 1997) is a Spanish adaptation of the National Adult Reading Test (NART) (Nelson and Willison, 1991) designed to estimate premorbid IQ by asking participants to correctly accentuate 30 low-frequency words with omitted accents. The test has shown strong psychometric properties, including high test–retest and inter-rater reliability, and good correlations with established intelligence measures such as the WAIS and Raven's Progressive Matrices. Normative data have been developed across multiple Spanish-speaking populations. In Spain, Del Pino et al. (2018) established normative data for the WAT in a large sample of 700 adults aged 18–86, stratified by both age (nine groups from 18–25 up to 81–86) and education. Their analyses showed that education accounted for a substantial proportion of the variance in WAT performance (33%), while age effects became apparent primarily from midlife onwards. Alternate forms were validated against pseudoword reading from the PROLEC-R, showing strong reliability and convergent validity. In Latin America, localized adaptations have strengthened the utility of the WAT. For example, the WAT, Buenos Aires, Argentina version (Burin et al, 2000) expanded the original list to 44 words, distributed across stress patterns (20% final syllable, 25% penultimate, 55% antepenultimate) and demonstrated excellent internal consistency (Cronbach's α = .94). Further work in Argentina and Colombia by Sierra et al. (2015) validated culturally appropriate versions in a sample of 240 adults (ages 20–74, evenly split between the two countries), with factor analyses confirming strong links between WAT performance and crystallized intelligence. Among Spanish-speaking immigrants in the U.S., Schrauf et al. (2006) adapted and validated a revised version in older adults (mean age 69.4 years, mean education 8.5 years), showing robust correlations with vocabulary and crystallized intelligence measures, including in bilingual participants, although age-related declines in performance were evident.

Strengths and Limitations: The Word Accentuation Test (WAT) shows strong reliability and validity, with high correlations to measures of crystallized intelligence (e.g., WAIS, Raven's Progressive Matrices) and consistent support across Spanish-speaking populations. Normative data from Spain (Del Pino et al, 2018), Latin America (Sierra Sanjurjo et al, 2015), and U.S. Spanish-speaking immigrants (Schrauf, Weintraub, and Navarro, 2006) provide age- and education-stratified norms, while local adaptations like the WAT-Buenos Aires demonstrate excellent internal consistency (α = .94). Strengths include its cultural adaptability and clinical utility in estimating premorbid IQ. Limitations involve uneven geographic representation, exclusion of illiterate individuals in some studies, and greater sensitivity to aging than pseudo-word reading tasks, which may reduce accuracy in older adults. Cross-national comparability also remains limited without harmonized norms.

Bateria Woodcock-Muñoz III Pruebas de Aprovechamiento (Subtest de Identificación de letras y palabras)

The Batería III Woodcock-Muñoz Pruebas de Aprovechamiento (Muñoz-Sandoval et al, 2005) is the Spanish adaptation of the WJ III, developed within the CHC theoretical framework to evaluate cognitive, linguistic, and academic abilities in Spanish speakers from ages 2–90. Subtests from the reading cluster, particularly word reading, reading comprehension, word decoding, reading fluency, and reading speed, are sometimes used to estimate premorbid cognitive ability. The WJ III was standardized on a large, geographically diverse U.S. sample covering ages 2–90+, and demonstrates strong psychometric properties, with reliabilities generally above .80 and often exceeding .90, meeting or surpassing accepted standards for individual placement and educational decision-making.

Strengths and Limitations: The Batería III Woodcock-Muñoz Pruebas de Aprovechamiento provides a reliable, theory-based assessment of cognitive and academic abilities in Spanish speakers with strong psychometrics and U.S. norms, though interpretation may be limited by cultural and dialectal differences and the generalizability of norms beyond the U.S.

ATTENTION

Visuospatial Span (Corsi's Test)

The Corsi block-tapping test, originally described by Milner and formalized by Corsi (1972), evaluates visuospatial short-term and working memory. In the forward version, participants reproduce the examiner's tapping sequence, while in the backward version, they repeat the sequence in reverse. The longest sequence correctly recalled is the "Corsi span," averaging 5–6 in typical adults (Kessels et al, 2000). Spanish norms were established in the NEURONORMA project using a sample of 349 participants from Spain (see pages 9–10 for more details on the NEURONORMA).

Digit Span (Forward and Backward)

Digit Span, first investigated by Jacobs, 1887 and later conceptualized by Miller, 1956 measures verbal short-term and working memory as well as attention. In its standard form, participants repeat digit sequences of increasing length either forward or backward. The WAIS Digit Span subtest is the most widely used format (Funes, Hernandez Rodriguez, and Lopez 2016; Inesta et al, 2021). Spanish norms are available in the WAIS-III manuals (Wechsler, 1987, 1997, 2003) (Artiola et al, 1999). More recently, the NEURONORMA project developed updated norms in a larger sample of 354 participants aged 50–90 (Pena-Casanova, Quinones-Ubeda et al, 2009)

Letter–Number Sequencing (WAIS-III, WAIS-IV)

This WAIS subtest measures short-term memory and mental manipulation by requiring participants to reorder mixed sequences of letters and numbers (numbers in ascending order, letters alphabetically). Spanish and Mexican adaptations are included in WAIS-III and WAIS-IV, with norms available through the NEURONORMA project. Receptive language demands influence performance, which is sensitive to age and education.

Arithmetic (WAIS-R)

The WAIS-R Arithmetic subtest assesses attention, concentration, working memory, mental manipulation, and numerical reasoning. The Spanish version mirrors the original WAIS-R procedures. The normative sample included 183 participants, with mean ages of 38.31 for women and 35.51 for men. Lower scores were associated with older age and fewer years of education.

Paced Auditory Serial Addition Test

The Paced Auditory Serial Addition Test (PASAT) measures attention, working memory, and processing speed by requiring participants to sum the two most recently presented digits at fixed intervals. In the NP-NUMBRS project, Spanish language norms were derived from 249 participants (58% female; mean age 37.3, range 19–60).

Brief Test of Attention

The Brief Test of Attention (BTA) evaluates auditory attention, working memory, sustained, and shifting attention, especially in the presence of competing stimuli (Schretlen, 1997). This test requires individuals to focus on and respond to specific target stimuli within a series of spoken numbers and letters. It is often used to identify attentional deficits in various populations, including those with brain injuries, neurological disorders, and attention-deficit/hyperactivity disorder (ADHD). In the U.S., Carrión et al. (2024) developed norms for the BTA in a sample of 245 Spanish-speaking adults aged 18–80 from eight states (California, Connecticut, Florida, Indiana, New Jersey, Oregon, Virginia, and Wisconsin). In that normative sample, BTA performance was found to increase as a function of increasing education. For normative data outside of the U.S., refer to Arango-Lasprilla (2015) norms under global measures for normative information, comprising a comprehensive set of neuropsychological tests designed to evaluate cognitive functions in Spanish-speaking populations. It includes various subtests to assess cognitive domains such as attention, memory, executive function, language, and visuospatial abilities.

Bells Test

The Bells Test is a cognitive assessment designed to evaluate selective attention and visual scanning abilities. It consists of 315 stimuli organized randomly on an 8½ × 11 sized sheet, divided into seven columns. Each column contains 45 stimuli, including 40 distractors and 5 target bells. Participants are asked to locate and mark the 35 bells among the 280 distractors.

Carrión et al. (2024) developed norms for the Bells Test in a sample of 245 Spanish-speaking adults aged 18–80 from eight states (California, Connecticut, Florida, Indiana, New Jersey, Oregon, Virginia, and Wisconsin). Their study revealed no significant influence of sociodemographic factors, including education, on test scores. Consequently, it appears unnecessary to make sociodemographic adjustments when utilizing the Bells Test with the U.S. Hispanic population.

"A" Cancellation Test

This measure is often used to assess attention, visual scanning abilities, and executive functioning, wherein participants are presented with a series of scattered letters on paper and asked to cross out every letter "A" as quickly as possible. Participants are timed, and the score is the number of correctly identified letter As. Norms for this test were derived from the larger battery by (Torres et al, 2021). This study includes sample characteristics and normative procedures for the larger sample. The sample size is unequal among all tests, as not all participants received the same battery. Notably, the "A" cancellation test was removed from the protocol due to psychometric limitations, resulting in fewer participants older than 33 with scores for this test.

Number Span Test

The objective of the Number Span Test (UDSv3) is to evaluate auditory attention, working memory, and sequential processing skills. There are two trials, one includes numbers forward and the other backward. The Spanish adaptation of the UDS3-NB involved preliminary translation and content review by expert clinicians and pilot testing at three U.S. and four Latin American sites. Refer to UDSv3 under global measures for details on sample characteristics and norms (Marquine et al, 2023).

Strengths and Limitations: These measures are widely used, easy to administer, and supported by Spanish language norms, making them valuable for assessing attention and executive control. Their standardized formats (e.g., Corsi, digit span, letter-number sequencing, arithmetic, PASAT) capture different cognitive processes and show good clinical utility. However, with the exception of the Bells test, performance is strongly influenced by age, education, and language, and some Spanish language norms are based on limited or uneven samples. Tasks like PASAT and Arithmetic may also be confounded by math skills or test anxiety, requiring cautious interpretation.

EXECUTIVE FUNCTIONS

Trail Making Test

The Trail Making Test (TMT) is a widely used measure of processing speed (Trails A) and executive functioning (Trails B) (Reitan, 1958). Normative data for Spanish-speaking populations have been developed across multiple regions. Arango-Lasprilla et al. (2015) created regression-based norms for 3,965 cognitively normal adults ages 18–95 from 11 Latin American countries, incorporating demographic predictors such as age, education, and gender. Suarez et al. (2021) extended this work with 252 adults ages 19–60 from the U.S.-Mexico border, adjusting for language preference, education, age, and gender using fractional polynomial regression. The language of the test was determined by a combination of the participants' self-reported language preferences (Spanish or English) and performance-based language fluency tests (Benton, 1994; Artiola i Fortuny, Heaton, and Hermosillo, 1998). In Colombia, Torres et al. (2021) norms for 2,673 adults (ages 18–86, with 1–25 years of education) were generated, stratified by age and education, with strict exclusion criteria to ensure cognitively normal status. This dataset also supported norms for additional executive measures, including the WCST and verbal fluency tasks. Together, these studies provide culturally relevant, regression-based norms for diverse Spanish-speaking populations, enhancing the TMT's clinical and research utility.

Using a novel Bayesian approach that takes into account language and acculturation, Carrión et al. (2024) demonstrated that for Spanish-speaking adults residing in the U.S., performance for TMT-A and TMT-B improved with higher education. This performance followed a logarithmic pattern, meaning that additional years of schooling led to faster completion times, particularly up to about 10 years of education. Age was also a key factor: older adults generally required more time to complete both parts of the test. For TMT-A, an additional interaction emerged between age and time living in the U.S., showing that individuals over 60 who had spent more years in the U.S. took longer to complete the test than those who had lived in the country for a shorter period. Overall, these findings suggest that education, age, and acculturation-related factors play significant roles in influencing processing speed and cognitive flexibility among Spanish-speaking individuals.

Strengths and Limitations: The TMT is a brief, widely validated measure of processing speed (Trails A) and executive functioning (Trails B) with regression-based normative data available for diverse Spanish-speaking populations, including large U.S. and Latin American samples (Arango-Lasprilla et al, 2015), U.S.-Mexico border cohorts (Suarez et al, 2021), and Colombian adults (Torres et al, 2021). These datasets enhance cultural relevance by incorporating demographic predictors such as age, education, gender, and language preference, and the Colombian norms also extend to related executive function tasks, supporting validity. However, comparability across studies is limited by differences in sample size, representativeness, and exclusion criteria, with some relying on MMSE cutoffs or self-report to define cognitive normality. Smaller regional samples, like those from the U.S.-Mexico border, further restrict generalizability, and performance may be influenced by literacy, motor speed, or cultural familiarity, which can complicate interpretation in lower-educated or older populations.

Symbol Digit Modalities Test

The Symbol Digit Modalities Test (SDMT) (Smith, 1973) is a digit–symbol substitution task that assesses divided attention, visual scanning and tracking, perceptual–motor speed, and working memory (Lezak, 2004). It can be administered in written or oral form, with strong construct validity across formats (Bowler, Thaler, and Rauch, 1992) and high test-retest reliability in healthy adults (0.84–0.93) (Benedict et al, 2012). The SDMT is sensitive to cognitive impairment, and performance is influenced by age and education (Strauss, Sherman, and Spreen, 2006; Ryan et al, 2020). Normative data for Spanish speakers were reported by Arango-Lasprilla et al. (2015), based on regression models explaining 29–55% of the variance in scores; sex was excluded as a predictor given its negligible effect size (<0.3). Among Spanish-speakers residing in the U.S., Carrión et al. (2024) found that performance on the SDMT, both oral and written versions, is influenced by complex interactions among age, education, sex, and Hispanic acculturation (BAS). Higher education, following a logarithmic pattern, was generally associated with better SDMT performance. However, age moderated these effects: younger individuals showed minimal differences, while older adults, especially those with lower education or lower Hispanic acculturation, tended to have lower scores. Interestingly, among those over age 30, higher Hispanic acculturation was linked to lower SDMT scores. For the written version, women outperformed men up to about 20 years of education, after which men scored higher. Overall, the results highlight that demographic and cultural factors, particularly education, age, and acculturation, interact in nuanced ways to influence attention and processing speed in Spanish-speaking populations.

Strengths and Limitations: The SDMT offers several strengths, including its brevity, ease of administration in both written and oral forms, and strong psychometric properties, with high test-retest reliability and good construct validity across administration modes. It is highly sensitive to cognitive impairment and widely used as a screening tool across clinical and research settings. Regression-based normative data for Spanish-speaking populations further enhance its applicability, accounting for demographic influences such as age and education. However, limitations include its susceptibility to demographic effects, particularly education and age, which can confound interpretation in diverse populations. The available normative data did not include sex as a predictor, which may overlook subtle differences, and the variance explained by regression models (29–55%) suggests other unmeasured factors may influence performance. Finally, while sensitive, the SDMT is not specific to particular cognitive domains, meaning impaired scores require follow-up with more targeted assessments.

The Wisconsin Card Sorting Test

The Wisconsin Card Sorting Test (WCST) is a neuropsychological test used to assess executive functions, particularly cognitive flexibility, problem-solving, and attention. The original test consists of 64 or 128 cards, each depicting a different combination of color, shape, and number of symbols (Heaton et al, 1993; Grant and Berg, 2014). The participant is asked to sort the cards into four piles based on a rule that they must discover through trial and error. The rule changes without warning after the participant has correctly sorted a certain number of cards (usually 10). The test continues until all cards have been sorted or a predetermined number of trials have been completed.

Marquine, Yassai-Gonzalez et al. (2021) developed normative data for the 64-item version of the Wisconsin Card Sorting Test (WCST-64) tailored for Spanish-speaking adults living in the U.S.-Mexico border region. The study included 189 native Spanish speakers (ages 19–60; education range: 0–20 years; 59.3% female) drawn from the Neuropsychological Norms for the U.S.-Mexico Border Region in Spanish (NP-NUMBRS) project. Fifty-nine participants were from Arizona and 130 from California. To examine the influence of demographic factors on performance, the authors analyzed univariable and interactive associations between age, education, gender, and raw WCST-64 scores using Spearman correlations, Wilcoxon rank-sum tests, and linear regressions. Demographically adjusted T-scores were generated for several key WCST-64 metrics, including total errors, perseverative responses, perseverative errors, conceptual-level responses, and number of categories, using fractional polynomial equations that accounted for age, education, and gender. Percentile scores were reported for the "Failures to Maintain Set" measure.

Findings showed that older age was associated with poorer performance, while higher education predicted better outcomes, particularly among female participants. The new norms produced expected impairment rates (14–16% across measures). When compared to existing norms, impairment rates based on norms for non-Hispanic Black adults were generally similar, while norms for non-Hispanic White adults overestimated impairment, with rates ranging from 38–52%.

Strengths and Limitations: Culturally tailored norms for a historically underrepresented group improve diagnostic accuracy in Spanish-speaking populations. Robust demographic modeling using regression-based approaches to adjust for age, education, and gender effects. The sample size is modest, coming from a specific region (the U.S.-Mexico border), which may limit generalizability to other Spanish-speaking populations in the U.S. or Latin America. Older adults (>60) were not included, restricting the applicability of these norms in aging or dementia-focused assessments. While education effects were examined, the study did not fully explore other sociocultural variables (e.g., SES, literacy, and acculturation) that may affect test performance.

The Modified Wisconsin Card Sorting Test

The Modified Wisconsin Card Sorting Test (M-WCST) (Nelson, 1976) is an adaptation of the original WCST, consisting of two sets of 24 response cards. Participants are notified when the sorting category changes and must adjust their approach, engaging abstract reasoning, feedback integration, cognitive flexibility, and inhibitory control (Zubicaray and Ashton, 1996). The M-WCST is sensitive to frontal lobe dysfunction across a range of conditions, including dementia, epilepsy, traumatic brain injury, and psychiatric disorders. Performance is influenced by demographic factors such as age, education, gender, and intellectual ability, with key outcomes including perseverative errors, categories achieved, and total errors. Spanish normative data have been reported by Arango-Lasprilla et al. (2015) (see the sample description on pages 8–9).

Strengths and Limitations: The M-WCST offers a shorter, more efficient alternative to the full WCST while maintaining sensitivity to executive dysfunction. It provides valuable indices of cognitive flexibility and error monitoring that are clinically relevant. However, demographic variables, particularly age and education, exert a strong influence on performance, which must be considered in interpretation. Within the Spanish normative database, sex was excluded as a predictor due to its negligible effect, and regression models explained a modest proportion of the variance (2–33% depending on outcome), suggesting that additional unmeasured factors contribute to performance. These limitations underscore the need for careful application and interpretation in diverse populations.

Verbal Fluency

Verbal Fluency Tasks are widely used measures of executive function that assess the rapid generation of words under phonological (e.g., letters FAS) or semantic (e.g., animals, fruits, clothing) constraints (Troyer, 2000; Strauss, Sherman, and Spreen, 2006; Thurstone, 1938). These tasks rely on cognitive flexibility, organization, inhibition, and sustained effort, and are sensitive to left frontal lobe dysfunction (Gouveia et al, 2007). Reliability is consistently strong, with internal consistency and test-retest values typically above .70–.80 (Tombaugh, Kozak, and Rees, 1999; Ruff et al, 1996). Demographic factors, including age, education, reading level, bilingualism, and intelligence shape performance.

Extensive normative data have been developed for Spanish-speaking populations. Rivera et al. (2019) reported norms for FAS and Animals in large cross-national samples, showing variance explained by age and education ranged from 7–43% across letters and categories, with gender excluded due to negligible effects. The sample description is presented on pages 8–9 (Guardia-Olmos et al, 2015). Verbal fluency tasks demonstrated strong psychometric properties, with internal reliability around .83 for both FAS (Tombaugh, Kozak, and Rees, 1999) and CFL (Ruff et al, 1996), and test-retest reliability typically exceeding .70 in healthy adults.

Chávez-Oliveros et al. (2015) generated normative data for the Semantic Verbal Fluency (Animals) test in Mexican adults aged 65 and older. The study included 1,233 cognitively healthy participants from both urban (Mexico City) and rural (State of Morelos) regions. Screening procedures involved the Community Screening Instrument for Dementia (CSI-D) and the Neuropsychiatric Inventory (NPI-Q), with exclusions for dementia or clinically significant depressive symptoms. Norms were derived using multiple linear regression and percentile scores, adjusted for demographic variables. Results showed that performance varied by age and education, with younger and more highly educated participants scoring higher. Mean scores were lower than in other studies, which the authors attributed to the lower educational attainment of the sample and the inclusion of participants over 100 years of age.

Rivera et al. (2019) extended this work by developing norms for Letter M, Fruits, and Occupations in a large sample of 3,977 adults (ages 18–95) from 10 Latin American countries and the U.S. (Argentina, Bolivia, Chile, Cuba, El Salvador, Guatemala, Honduras, Mexico, Paraguay, Peru, and Puerto Rico). All participants were born and residing in their respective countries, had at least one year of formal education, and the norms incorporated country-specific adjustments for age, education, and gender. Rodríguez-Lorenzana et al. (2020) established phonological (F, A, S, M) and semantic (animals, fruits) norms for 322 Ecuadorian adults from Quito, adjusting for age, education, and gender. Multiple linear regression models examined the impact of demographic variables on test performance.

Olabarrieta-Landa et al. (2024) recently established U.S.-based norms for verbal fluency tests, including phonological (letters F, A, S, P, M, and R) and semantic (animals, fruits) tasks, using a sample of 245 Spanish-speaking adults aged 18–80 from eight states (California, Connecticut, Florida, Indiana, New Jersey, Oregon, Virginia, and Wisconsin). A Bayesian approach was applied to account for sociocultural and linguistic factors, with eligibility requiring Spanish fluency and at least one year of U.S. residence.

Strengths and Limitations: Verbal fluency tasks are brief, reliable measures of executive functioning that are sensitive to frontal lobe dysfunction and widely used across Spanish-speaking populations. Large normative datasets from Latin America, Mexico, Ecuador, and the U.S. provide culturally relevant reference values, often adjusted for age, education, and sometimes gender or language use.

Their strengths lie in ease of administration, strong psychometric properties, and broad applicability, but limitations include variability in sample representativeness, inconsistent use of demographic predictors, and cross-study differences in letter or category selection. Specifically, while FAS is standard for English speakers with letter choice based on word frequency per letter, PMR may be a better option as it was adapted to ensure comparable word frequency difficulty per letter and minimize cultural bias for Spanish speakers. Performance is also strongly shaped by age and education, which may limit comparability and generalizability across diverse groups. While Olabarrieta-Landa et al. (2024) norms enhance the cultural and linguistic relevance of assessments for U.S. Spanish speakers, the sample's relatively high educational level may limit generalizability to populations with more diverse educational backgrounds.

Stroop Color Word Test

Since its development in 1935, the Stroop Color-Word Test has undergone multiple revisions to vary its stimuli and administration (Golden, Freshwater, and Golden, 1978). It remains a core executive function measure, tapping selective attention, cognitive flexibility, inhibition, and processing speed (Strauss, Sherman, and Spreen, 2006). Early normative work included individuals aged 5–90, with adequate test-retest reliability on the interference trial. In Golden, Freshwater, and Golden (1978), Spanish adaptation, reliabilities were strong for Word (.89), Color (.84), and Color-Word (.73) trials. Interference scores correlated with other inhibition tasks (e.g., stop-signal), demonstrated sensitivity to executive dysfunction, and have been widely applied in clinical populations (Scarpina and Tagini, 2017). Performance is known to vary with age, education, and practice effects.

In Latin America, Rivera, Perrin, Stevens et al. (2015) provided normative data for 3,977 healthy adults across 11 countries (Argentina, Bolivia, Chile, Cuba, El Salvador, Guatemala, Honduras, Mexico, Paraguay, Peru, and Puerto Rico, U.S.), showing consistent age-related declines and education-related improvements, particularly for those with more than 12 years of education. Country-specific patterns emerged, with some variability in Word-Color performance across sites. In Spain, the NEURONORMA study (Pena-Casanova, Blesa et al, 2009) generated norms for 344 adults aged 50–90, adjusting scores for both age and education. In the U.S., Ramos Usuga et al. (2024) established regression-based norms for 245 Spanish speakers across eight states (California, Connecticut, Florida, Indiana, New Jersey, Oregon, Virginia, and Wisconsin). Using a Bayesian approach, they observed linear declines with age, education effects after 15 years, and notable influences of sex and Spanish proficiency. For example, women with higher Spanish proficiency outperformed men, and bilinguals with balanced proficiency performed consistently across education levels. Stroop Color-Word and interference scores also showed age-related decline but improved with higher education and greater Spanish proficiency.

Strengths and Limitations: These studies highlight the value of regression-based approaches and replicate patterns observed in English-speaking samples, where age and education strongly predict performance. However, the norms are specific to the populations studied and cannot be assumed to generalize beyond those cultural and regional contexts.

Raven's Progressive Matrices

The Raven's Progressive Matrices (RPM) is a widely used nonverbal measure of abstract reasoning and fluid intelligence, assessing pattern recognition and problem-solving with minimal reliance on language or cultural knowledge. Its versatility has made it valuable in neuropsychological, clinical, educational, and forensic contexts (Sherman, Tan, and Hrabok, 2023).

The test exists in three original forms: the Colored Progressive Matrices (CPM) for children (5.5+ years) and individuals with neurological or cognitive impairments; the Standard Progressive Matrices (SPM) for the general population (6.5+ years); and the Advanced Progressive Matrices (APM) for adolescents and adults with above-average abilities (Raven, 1938; Raven, 1995; Raven, 2000).

The Raven's 2: Second Edition and its Spanish adaptation (Raven, 2019) represent the most recent updates. Available in paper and digital formats, these versions provide age-specific short and long forms, updated stimuli, improved standardization, and automated scoring via Pearson's Q-global system. Norms span ages 4 to 69 years and 11 months. Digital delivery reduces memorization effects by randomly drawing items from a larger bank while maintaining high equivalence with paper forms (r = .93). Unlike earlier RPM versions, Raven's 2 employs colored designs to enhance engagement (Sherman, Tan, and Hrabok, 2023). Across versions, the RPM demonstrates strong psychometric properties. Split-half reliability coefficients typically exceed .80, and test-retest reliability remains above .80 for short intervals. Construct validity is well established: the RPM aligns with Spearman's concept of general intelligence factor (the g-factor), which represents an individual's overall cognitive capability. The RPM also correlates with other nonverbal measures such as the Kaufman Brief Intelligence Test Second Edition (KBIT-2), and shows appropriate convergent, divergent, and criterion validity across populations (Carpenter, Just, and Shell, 1990; Bors and Stokes, 1998).

Strengths and Limitations: The RPM has notable strengths, including its nonverbal design, broad applicability across age and ability levels, and strong reliability and validity as a measure of fluid intelligence. Updated versions, such as Raven's 2, improve accessibility with digital formats and regression-based norms. However, performance is still influenced by factors like age, education, and cultural exposure, meaning the test is not entirely culture-free. The availability and quality of localized norms can also limit cross-cultural comparability.

Working Memory Index

The Working Memory Index (WMI) is a score obtained from specific subtests of the WAIS-III and WAIS-IV. It reflects an individual's capacity to focus on verbally presented information, hold and manipulate it in short-term memory, and use it to generate an appropriate response. For the WAIS-III, Arithmetic, Digit Span, and Letter–Number Sequencing serve as the core subtests that make up the WMI. In the WAIS-IV, the index is calculated using Arithmetic and Digit Span as the primary subtests, with Letter–Number Sequencing included only as an optional supplemental measure.

LANGUAGE

Boston Naming Test

The Boston Naming Test (BNT) is a widely used measure of word retrieval that uses black-and-white line drawings to elicit object names. Originally developed with 85 items (Kaplan, Goodglass, and Weintraub, 1978), it was later standardized into a 60-item version, with a 15-item short form created to reduce administration time (Lansing et al, 1999). Word retrieval requires sequential perceptual recognition of the stimulus followed by activation of semantic and phonological systems; processes linked to Broca's area, Wernicke's area, and adjacent regions in both hemispheres. While clinically valuable, the validity of the BNT has been questioned due to item-specific cultural and linguistic differences that may complicate interpretation across diverse populations (Marquez de la Plata et al, 2009; Loewenstein et al, 1994).

Several studies have established norms for Spanish-speaking populations. As part of the Neuropsychological Screening Battery for Hispanics (NeSBHIS; n = 300 bilingual and monolingual Spanish speakers aged 16–75), Ponton et al. (1996) provided normative data for a 30-item version of the BNT (Pontón-Satz BNT), and removed items deemed to the be culturally biased for Hispanics including "pretzel," "igloo," "acorn," and "trellis." In this normative sample, males were found to outperform females, and BNT scores were positively associated with education. The project FRONTIER study (n = 380, ages 40–96) similarly included a version of the BNT; however, this was a Spanish-English equivalent version developed using item-response theory (Jahn et al, 2013). Jahn et al. (2013) found that out of the original items, 27 showed differential item functioning (DIF), meaning they did not measure naming ability equivalently between English and Spanish speakers. The resulting 15-item version effectively balances difficulty and discrimination, offering a valid and efficient tool for assessing confrontation naming in bilingual and monolingual populations. These results emphasize that the full BNT may not provide valid assessments for Spanish speakers due to linguistic and cultural differences in item difficulty, and they support using the brief version to ensure fair comparisons across language groups. Olabarrieta-Landa et al. (2015) developed norms for the 60-item BNT across 11 Latin American countries using a large sample of 3,779 individuals aged 10–95, with adjustments for age, sex, and education. Olabarrieta-Landa et al. (2015) provided Costa Rican norms for the 15-item BNT in 563 healthy older adults (ages 59–90), demonstrating education and sex effects on performance and creating a calculator to generate demographically adjusted scores. In Spain, Peña-Casanova et al. (2009) published norms for 340 cognitively normal participants aged 50–94 from multiple regions, adapting culturally sensitive items (e.g., replacing "pretzel" with "magdalena") and employing an overlapping interval strategy to optimize age distributions. Finally, the BNT-15 is included in the CERAD battery, with norms described in Fillenbaum et al. (2007) and Torres et al. (2021).

Strengths and Limitations: The BNT is a widely used and valuable measure of word retrieval with strong neuroanatomical correlates, making it an essential tool in the assessment of language and cognitive disorders. Its strengths include extensive clinical use, availability in multiple versions (60-, 30-, and 15-item forms), and the development of normative data for diverse Spanish-speaking populations across Latin America, Spain, and the U.S., often adjusted for age, sex, and education. However, the BNT's validity can be compromised by linguistic and cultural differences, as some items may not translate equivalently or hold the same relevance across populations, potentially leading to misinterpretation. The test is also sensitive to education and bilingualism, factors not always fully accounted for in earlier normative studies, which limits generalizability when norms are applied outside their original contexts.

The current study improves upon these limitations by using item response theory (IRT) to identify and remove items that function differently across English and Spanish versions, resulting in a 15-item bilingual BNT with demonstrated psychometric equivalence. This approach enhances cross-linguistic validity, reduces cultural bias, and offers a more accurate measure of naming ability for both English- and Spanish-speaking individuals. Nonetheless, further research is needed to establish diagnostic accuracy and normative data for the new 15-item version across clinical and cultural subgroups.

The Texas Spanish Naming Test

The Texas Spanish Naming Test (TNT) was developed specifically in Spanish to reduce cultural and linguistic bias, consisting of 30 object drawings presented in order of difficulty (Marquez de la Plata et al, 2008). It was validated in 85 older Hispanic adults from two Primary Care Clinics in Dallas, Texas; most were Mexican-born and Spanish-dominant, and all were 65 years of age and older. The TNT showed diagnostic utility in distinguishing dementia from non-dementia groups when compared to other Spanish naming tests.

Strengths and Limitations: The TNT offers the strength of being developed directly in Spanish to minimize cultural and linguistic bias, with evidence of diagnostic utility in distinguishing dementia from non-dementia groups. However, its limitations include reliance on vocabulary derived from Spaniard participants that may not reflect broader Spanish usage, and a validation sample composed largely of older, Mexican-origin individuals, reducing generalizability to other Spanish-speaking populations.

Multilingual Naming Test

The Multilingual Naming Test (MINT) consists of 68 black-and-white drawings presented in order of increasing difficulty and was developed for Spanish, English, Mandarin, and Hebrew speakers. To minimize cultural and linguistic bias, cognates were excluded, as were items with multiple acceptable names or those disproportionately difficult in one language compared to others (Gollan et al, 2012). Validation studies included 112 young adults (monolingual and Spanish-English bilinguals) and 20 older bilinguals from UCSD's Alzheimer's Disease Research Center's (ADRC) cohort, with language dominance and index scores calculated to capture differences between bilinguals. The MINT demonstrated sensitivity to naming deficits and language dominance, offering a more culturally balanced alternative to the BNT, which has notable linguistic and cultural limitations (Weintraub et al, 2018b). More recently, Marquine et al. (2023) published Spanish-language norms for the UDS 3, including the MINT, in U.S. Latinos aged 50–94, adjusting for age, sex, and education. Results showed education was the strongest predictor of performance, particularly among Spanish-speakers, who generally scored lower than English-speakers even after demographic adjustments, highlighting the impact of cultural and linguistic context. Importantly, derived intraindividual comparison scores were less affected by demographics, suggesting a fairer approach to diagnosis across diverse populations. A normative calculator is also available through the NACC website to facilitate clinical use.

Strengths and Limitations: The MINT offers clear strengths as a culturally sensitive alternative to the BNT, with careful item selection to minimize language bias and proven utility in detecting naming deficits, including in Alzheimer's disease. Its inclusion in the UDS3 and the development of Spanish language norms tailored for U.S. Latinos (Marquine et al, 2023) enhance its clinical applicability and equity in multilingual assessments. Limitations include reliance on relatively small, homogeneous validation samples, strong demographic influences (age, education, and language dominance), and lower performance among Spanish-speakers even after adjustment. While valuable, broader validation across more diverse populations is still needed.

Token Test

The Token Test (TT), (De Renzi and Vignolo, 1962), is a widely used measure of oral comprehension, syntax, and working memory. Originally developed for adults with aphasia, it has since been applied across diverse populations, including individuals with receptive disorders, various types of aphasia, learning disorders, and dementia. Over time, several adaptations have been introduced, such as the abbreviated Token Test (aTT) with 36 simplified commands and modified colors to reduce visual discrimination issues, short and computerized versions, and integration into batteries like the Multilingual Aphasia Examination (Benton, Hamsher, and Sivan, 1994).

More recently, normative data for Spanish speakers have been broadened. Julio-Ramos et al. (2024) developed norms for the Spanish abbreviated Token Test (Sp-aTT) using a sample of 210 healthy adults and 197 stroke patients in Chile, after careful cultural and linguistic adaptation. Results showed excellent diagnostic accuracy (AUC = 0.97) and highlighted education as a more influential factor than age, leading to cutoff adjustments. Norms were derived through linear models accounting for age, education, and their interaction with group type.

Pena-Casanova et al. (2009) also published norms for Spain using a 36-item short form, while Rey et al, 1999 established norms for Spanish as part of the Multilingual Aphasia Examination (MAE) standardization.

Strengths and Limitations: The TT's strengths lie in its sensitivity to subtle receptive language deficits, adaptability across languages and populations, and its robust psychometric validation, including high diagnostic accuracy in clinical groups. However, performance is strongly influenced by education, which complicates interpretation in low-literacy populations, and current Spanish norms are restricted to specific countries (e.g., Chile and Spain), limiting generalizability across diverse Spanish-speaking communities.

Multilingual Aphasia Examination

Benton's Multilingual Aphasia Examination (MAE) marked one of the earliest attempts to standardize aphasia assessment across languages, prioritizing careful item selection, large stratified normative samples, and cross-linguistic validation (Benton, 1967; Benton, Hamsher, and Sivan, 1983). Within this framework, the TT became central because of its sensitivity to receptive language impairments. Rey et al. (1999) produced the Spanish adaptation, emphasizing cultural and linguistic appropriateness rather than literal translation. Adjustments included pilot testing across Hispanic subgroups, consulting the Real Academia de la Lengua Española for lexical accuracy, and refining items to preserve difficulty levels while ensuring cultural relevance.

The Spanish MAE (MAE-S) was normed on 234 Spanish-speaking adults aged 18–70, with no neurological history, stratified by sex, age, and education (<4 years, 5–7, 8–11, 12–15, 16+). In addition, preliminary norms were reported for 75 Spanish speakers on other Benton neuropsychological measures (e.g., Judgment of Line Orientation, Facial Recognition, Visual Form Discrimination, Temporal Orientation). Statistical analyses included t-tests, MANOVAs, and Bonferroni corrections to compare subgroups (e.g., Puerto Rican versus Mexican) and to benchmark Hispanic participants' performance against established U.S. English-speaking norms (Benton, Hamsher, and Sivan, 1983). Median scores, cutoff points, and standard deviations were computed for each test. Importantly, demographic influences such as age, sex, and education were incorporated into regression models, with education exerting the strongest effect. Results demonstrated a high degree of correspondence between Spanish-speaking participants' scores and English-based standards, supporting concurrent validity. Criterion validity was further established in clinical samples (e.g., dementia, stroke, head injury), which showed the adapted measures could reliably detect receptive language impairments in Spanish-speaking adults.

Strengths and Limitations: The adaptation ensured linguistic equivalence while maintaining standardized difficulty, allowing for valid cross-linguistic comparisons. Rigorous pilot work and stratified norms enhanced both cultural sensitivity and diagnostic accuracy. However, the normative sample was geographically limited and skewed toward higher educational attainment, reducing generalizability to less-educated or rural Spanish-speaking populations. Broader sampling across Latin America and among bilingual speakers remains a key gap for strengthening the clinical utility of the MAE-S.

Boston Diagnostic Aphasia Examination, Third Edition

The Boston Diagnostic Aphasia Examination (BDAE), developed by Goodglass and Kaplan (Goodglass and Kaplan, 1972) revised in 1983 (Goodglass and Kaplan, 1983), and revised again in 2001 (Goodglass, Kaplan, and Barresi, 2001), is a comprehensive assessment of language functions across auditory, visual, gestural, and written modalities. A Spanish adaptation was first introduced in Argentina (Cuschnir and Faiman, 1979), with a second edition in 1986 that corrected translation errors, refined scoring (e.g., replacing Z-scores with percentiles), and adjusted the paraphasia profile (Pineda et al, 2000).

Normative studies in Colombia established culturally appropriate benchmarks: Rosselli et al. (1990) tested 180 Spanish speakers from Bogotá using a 2 × 3 × 3 factorial design (sex × age × education). Participants were stratified into sex (male/female), three age groups (16–30, 31–50, and 51–65), and three education groups (0–5, 6–12, and 13+ years). All participants were screened for neurological and psychiatric conditions, ensuring a cognitively healthy sample. Results emphasized education as the strongest predictor of BDAE performance, with low-education individuals performing within ranges often seen in brain-damaged populations, highlighting the risk of misclassification without education-adjusted norms.

Building on this, Pineda et al. (2000) validated the 1986 Spanish BDAE in 156 native Spanish speakers from Medellín, stratified by age (19–35, 36–50, and 51–60), education (1–9, 10–15, and >16 years), socioeconomic status, and occupation. The adaptation included culturally appropriate lexical changes (e.g., "goma" → "caucho," "Sevilla" → "Bogotá") and excluded universally easy items to improve sensitivity. Administration was standardized through trained speech pathology students, with supervision to ensure inter-rater reliability. Factor analysis revealed seven components, with reading and writing domains explaining most of the variance, confirming the test's construct validity in Spanish. Again, education emerged as the most significant predictor of test performance, while age had modest effects, and sex, SES, and occupation showed minimal direct influence. These findings reinforce the importance of education-adjusted cutoffs and culturally adapted items for accurate interpretation of BDAE scores in Spanish-speaking populations. Together, these normative studies provided a robust foundation for the clinical and research use of the BDAE across Latin America and U.S. Spanish speakers, where standardized aphasia measures were previously lacking.

Strengths and Limitations: The Spanish adaptations of the BDAE offer a comprehensive tool for evaluating aphasia, with strengths including careful cultural and linguistic modifications (e.g., item substitutions for Colombian Spanish), standardized administration, and normative data stratified by age, sex, education, and socioeconomic factors. Validation studies confirmed strong construct validity, particularly in reading and writing domains, and highlighted the test's clinical utility in differentiating aphasic from non-aphasic individuals. However, limitations remain: the strongest predictor of performance is education, meaning low-education individuals may appear impaired without education-adjusted cutoffs. In addition, most validation samples came from urban Colombian populations, which may reduce generalizability to rural or other Spanish-speaking groups across Latin America and the U.S.

VERBAL MEMORY

Wechsler Memory Scale IV—Escala de Memoria Wechsler, Versión España IV

The Spanish version of the Wechsler Memory Scale IV (WMS-IV) was culturally adapted for tests that required more than simple translation (Logical Memory and Verbal Paired Associates). The cultural adaptation process took place in a pilot study with 50 individuals (50% female) with a median age of 38.1 years (Wechsler, 2009).

Logical Memory Subtest

The Logical Memory subtest assesses immediate recall, delayed recall, and recognition of short stories. In Spain, normative data were first established from a large census-based sample of 810 adults aged 16–89, stratified by age, sex, education, and geographic region, with norms derived using polynomial regression methods available in the WMS manual (Wechsler, 2009). Brugulat-Serrat et al. (2021) extended this work by providing biomarker-based norms for 248 middle-aged adults (50–70 years) from the ALFA+ cohort, using regression-based equations adjusted for age, education, and sex. Campos-Magdaleno et al. (2024) provided complementary data from 736 community-dwelling adults from Madrid, aged 50–88, stratified by education and age, generating adjusted scaled scores through linear regression and excluding individuals with depression or cognitive impairment. In the U.S., O'Bryant et al. (2018) created regression-based norms for 653 Mexican Americans from two Texas-based studies (Texas Alzheimer's research and care consortium; and health and Aging Brain Latino elders), both Spanish and English speakers, age 40+, stratifying scores by age and education bands following the Mayo method; education showed the strongest effect, with cutoffs adjusted for 0–6, 3–9, 6–12, and >12 years of schooling.

Strengths and Limitations: Strengths include large, well-characterized Spanish samples and the use of regression-based methods that account for demographic variables, with the ALFA+ cohort adding validation against AD biomarkers. The Mexican American study broadened applicability to U.S. Latino populations, though language dominance was not controlled. Limitations include restricted cultural representation (primarily Spain and Mexican Americans) and strong education effects that complicate interpretation in groups with less formal education. Together, these norms improve the test's clinical utility but highlight the need for broader cross-cultural validation.

Verbal Paired Associates Subtest

The Verbal Paired Associates (VPA; Pares de palabras) assesses explicit verbal episodic memory by presenting word pairs that participants must recall when cued with the first word. The Spanish adaptation considered word frequency, length, and difficulty, structuring the first four items as semantically related and the remaining six as unrelated. The adult version includes 14 pairs, while the older adult version uses 10 pairs. Normative data are available in the WMS manual (see Wechsler, 2009).

Strengths and Limitations: The VPA offers a structured assessment of associative learning and verbal episodic memory, with adaptations in Spanish that account for word frequency, length, and semantic relatedness, making it more culturally appropriate. Its inclusion of both related and unrelated word pairs allows for a nuanced evaluation of memory strategies and error patterns. However, limitations include reliance on culturally specific vocabulary, which may reduce comparability across diverse Spanish-speaking populations, and the lack of extensive normative data beyond the WMS manual, particularly for Latin American samples.

Craft Story

The Craft Story (CS), developed by Craft et al. (1996) is a widely used measure of verbal narrative memory included in the NACC Uniform Data Set (UDSv3). It assesses encoding, retention, and recall of complex information through immediate and delayed story recall, with scoring that captures both verbatim (max = 44) and paraphrased recall (max = 25), providing a nuanced profile of memory ability.

The CS was incorporated into the Spanish translation of UDSv3 in 2017 (Acevedo et al, 2009). Translation and adaptation involved expert review and pilot testing across U.S. and Latin American sites. While most neuropsychological tests required minimal changes, the CS underwent specific cultural and linguistic modifications to ensure appropriateness for Spanish-speaking populations. To support accurate interpretation, Alzheimer's Disease

Centers also began collecting a Linguistic History Form to document participants' language background and acculturation. As part of the UDSv3 Spanish-language normative study (N = 437; ages 50–94), Marquine et al. (2023) reported that education was the strongest predictor of performance on the CS 21 task for both English- and Spanish-speaking participants. Among English speakers, female sex was additionally associated with better performance on Craft Immediate Recall, whereas this sex-related advantage was not observed among Spanish speakers.

Strengths and Limitations: The CS provides a nuanced evaluation of verbal episodic memory by scoring both verbatim and paraphrased recall, which increases sensitivity to subtle memory deficits and supports its use in dementia research and clinical settings. The Spanish adaptation followed a careful translation and review process, with added attention to cultural and linguistic appropriateness, and the inclusion of a Linguistic History Form allows examiners to consider bilingualism and acculturation when interpreting results. Nonetheless, the adaptation relied on relatively small pilot samples, and normative data remain limited for Spanish speakers across diverse regions. Dialectal differences, variations in education, and cultural familiarity with the story content may still influence performance, highlighting the need for broader validation and more representative norms across U.S. Latino and Latin American populations.

Spanish English Verbal Learning Test

The Spanish-English Verbal Learning Test (SEVLT) was specifically designed to assess episodic memory in Latino/Hispanic populations and can be administered in either English or Spanish, with direct translations of test items. It uses a 15-word list drawn from five semantic categories (vegetables, drinks, kitchen utensils, reading materials, and one fruit) presented across five learning trials, followed by an interference list and an immediate post-interference recall trial (González et al, 2001). Initial normative data were based on 689 adults aged 60 and older, predominantly of Mexican ancestry (88.2%), recruited through community surveys in California. Additionally, participants had to self-identify as Hispanic or Latino, and bilingual participants chose the language in which they wanted to be tested. Regression-based norms adjusting for age, education, and gender were developed, though the potential inclusion of individuals with dementia may have inflated variability. To address this, additional analyses excluded cases scoring below the 10th percentile on an education- and age-adjusted MMSE, producing more conservative reference values.

A subsequent re-norming (González, Mungas, and Haan, 2002) expanded the sample to 1,686 older adults, again mostly of Mexican ancestry, and explicitly excluded individuals with dementia using clinical diagnostic criteria (NINCDS/ADRDA for AD and California ADTC criteria for ischemic vascular dementia). Regression equations were developed to adjust scores for demographics, and percentile cutoffs were provided for clinical use. Importantly, bilingual participants were allowed to choose their test language, and correct responses were accepted in either English or Spanish, reducing linguistic bias.

To extend generalizability, the Brief SEVLT (B-SEVLT) was implemented as part of the Hispanic Community Health Study/Study of Latinos (HCHS/SOL), a large, multisite cohort of 9,309 participants aged 45 and older, representing diverse Hispanic/Latino groups (Central American, Cuban, Dominican, Mexican American, Puerto Rican, and South American) (Breton et al, 2021). This version uses three learning trials instead of five, and normative data were derived using survey-adjusted regression models. Norms were stratified by age, sex, education, language of administration, and heritage group. A publicly available dashboard was also developed to generate standardized scores, offering clinicians a practical tool for applying these norms. Validation analyses confirmed that higher education, younger age, and female sex were associated with better performance, while significant differences emerged across heritage groups, underscoring the need for demographic-specific interpretation.

Strengths and Limitations: The SEVLT and B-SEVLT are valuable because they were developed and normed specifically for Hispanic/Latino populations, with large, diverse samples and demographic adjustments for age, education, sex, and heritage. Accepting responses in either Spanish or English also improves fairness for bilinguals. Limitations include the absence of a delayed recall trial, possible inclusion of dementia cases in early norms, and reliance on self-reported health status. While the B-SEVLT broadens representation, cultural and linguistic variability across Hispanic groups still limits generalizability, making subgroup-specific norms essential.

Hopkins Verbal Learning Test-Revised

The Hopkins Verbal Learning Test-Revised (HVLT-R) is a list-learning measure of verbal memory, modeled after the California Verbal Learning Test (CVLT), with six alternate forms and an added delayed recall trial. Performance is influenced by age, sex, education, and ethnicity (Benedict et al, 1998). Early U.S.-Mexico border norms (Cherner et al, 2007) highlighted inadequacies of the original norms for individuals with low education, leading to Spanish adaptations using careful translation, back-translation, and culturally neutral vocabulary reviewed by experts from multiple Spanish-speaking countries. Regression-based, education-adjusted scaled scores and percentiles were derived from 127 Spanish-speaking adults (ages 20–55 and 0–20 years of education). Broader norms for Latin American Spanish speakers were later developed by Arango-Lasprilla et al. (2015) using 3,972 adults (ages 18–95) from 11 countries, though these exclude illiterate individuals and may not generalize beyond the sampled regions. This normative study used version 5 of the HVLT-R (professions, sports, and vegetables). Region-specific norms include NP-NUMBRS (Díaz-Santos et al, 2020), based on 201 Spanish speakers (ages 19–60 and 0–20 years of education) from the U.S.-Mexico border, with regression-based T-scores adjusted for age, sex, and education, improving diagnostic accuracy but limited to that population. In Spain, Sáez-Atxukarro et al. (2021) provided norms from 700 adults (ages 18–90 and 0–25 years of education) through the Normacog Project, adjusting primarily for age and education.

Strengths and Limitations: The HVLT-R offers strong cultural and linguistic adaptations, with norms developed for Spanish speakers in Mexico, Latin America, Spain, and the U.S.-Mexico border, enhancing its validity across diverse groups. These norms adjust for key demographics like age, education, and sex, improving diagnostic accuracy. However, their applicability is limited by sample restrictions (e.g., NP-NUMBRS only for ages 19–60 and ≤20 years of education), exclusion of illiterate individuals, and reliance on brief screeners rather than full diagnostic evaluations. Clinicians must therefore select norms carefully to match the individual's background.

Memory Capacity Test

The Memory Capacity Test (MCT) (Buschke, 1984) is an associative memory task adapted for Spanish speakers in Antioquia, Colombia (Romero Vanegas et al, 2010). It uses two 16-item lists across semantic categories, with paired cued recall trials followed by free recall. Norms were later established in a large Colombian sample n = 2,673 (Torres et al, 2021) stratified by age and education, showing small effects of these variables and no effect of sex. The test has demonstrated sensitivity to preclinical and clinical memory decline in PSEN1 E280A mutation carriers.

Strengths and Limitations: The MCT is a culturally adapted tool that effectively measures associative memory and has shown strong clinical sensitivity in differentiating PSEN1 mutation carriers from controls, with large normative data available stratified by age and education. However, its norms are limited to Colombian samples, with skewed age distribution and broad education groupings, which restricts generalizability to other Spanish-speaking populations.

The World Health Organization, University of California, Los Angeles, Auditory Verbal Learning Test

The World Health Organization, University of California, Los Angeles (WHO-UCLA) Auditory Verbal Learning Test (WHO-UCLA AVLT) was developed in 1993 through a collaboration between the WHO and UCLA to provide a culturally fair measure of verbal learning and memory, using semantically grouped words from universally recognizable categories (body parts, animals, tools, household objects, vehicles) (Maj et al, 1993). Modeled after the Rey Auditory Verbal Learning Test (RAVLT), it includes five immediate recall trials, an interference list, short- and long-delay recall, and recognition, offering a comprehensive profile of encoding, retention, and retrieval processes. After the WHO-UCLA AVLT was created, it was integrated into the Neuropsychological Screening Battery for Hispanics (NeSBHIS) (Ponton et al, 1996).

Normative data for Spanish-speaking Hispanic adults in the U.S. were recently published by Arango-Lasprilla et al. (2024). Their sample included 245 adults (ages 18–80) recruited across eight states, all native Spanish speakers with ≥1 year of formal education, preserved cognitive status (MMSE ≥ 23), and no psychiatric, neurological, or substance-use history. Validation analyses revealed clear demographic effects: education strongly influenced all trials except recognition, with gains up to about 13 years before leveling off; age effects were smaller but present; and acculturation, indexed by longer U.S. residency, was associated with worse total recall, possibly reflecting decreased Spanish use. A notable interaction showed women with higher Spanish proficiency outperforming men on long-delay recall. Importantly, norms were generated using regression-based methods, yielding percentile ranks and an online calculator that adjusts for age, sex, education, and years in the U.S., increasing clinical applicability.

Strengths and Limitations: The WHO-UCLA AVLT is a culturally sensitive measure of verbal learning and memory, with strengths including neutral word lists, a comprehensive design, and new Spanish norms with an online calculator that adjusts for demographics and acculturation. These features enhance its clinical utility for U.S. Hispanic populations. However, the normative sample was relatively small, skewed toward educated middle-aged women, and validation across more diverse Hispanic subgroups is still needed to improve generalizability.

NEUROPSI Atención y Memoria, Word List/Stories

The Word-List test of the NEUROPSI (Ostrosky-Solis et al, 2007) involves three learning trials of 12 words drawn from three semantic categories (animals, fruits, and body parts), with performance scored as the average number of words recalled across trials. After a 20-minute delay, participants complete a free recall, followed by a cued recall based on category. A recognition trial then requires identifying the 12 target words among 24 items, including semantically and phonemically related distractors, with errors such as intrusions, perseverations, and false positives recorded. The Logical Memory subtests (I and II) complement this by assessing narrative memory, with participants recalling two short stories immediately (LM I) and again after a 20-minute delay (LM II). The NEUROPSI was standardized in Mexico, with normative data available (see pages 20–21) that incorporate adjustments for age, education, and other demographic variables. These norms enhance the test's diagnostic accuracy and ensure its clinical usefulness for diverse populations.

Strengths and Limitations: The NEUROPSI Atención y Memoria's main strength is its cultural and linguistic adaptation for Mexican populations, with norms adjusted for age and education that enhance diagnostic accuracy. However, its applicability is limited outside Mexico, as cultural and educational differences in other Spanish-speaking groups may affect performance, highlighting the need for broader validation.

Spanish Verbal Selective Reminding Task

The Verbal Selective Reminding Test (vSRT), as adapted by Campo, Morales, and Juan-Malpartida (2000), evaluates associative learning and memory through repeated recall, cued recall, and recognition trials. Campo and Morales (2004) provided normative data for Form 1 in 329 Spanish adults aged 18–59, stratified by age, sex, and education, and also examined alternate form reliability in a separate sample of 263 participants. Analyses confirmed the influence of age and education, with Bonferroni corrections applied to multiple comparisons, and alternate forms showed good reliability. Morales et al. (2010) expanded norms to 884 neurologically healthy adults aged 15–93, stratified into seven age cohorts and three education levels, with regression models confirming that age and education were the strongest predictors, and women generally outperformed men. These norms broadened applicability across adulthood and into older age, with correlations supporting test–retest reliability and form equivalence.

Strengths and limitations: The vSRT has strong psychometric properties, with test-retest and alternate form reliability and robust norms stratified by age, sex, and education, including large samples spanning ages 15–93. These features make it valuable for assessing learning and memory across adulthood. However, its norms come primarily from Spanish populations, limiting generalizability to U.S. Latinos or other Spanish-speaking groups, and data for the very old remain scarce.

The Free and Cued Selective Reminding Test

The Free and Cued Selective Reminding Test (FCSRT) is designed to assess episodic memory by combining free recall with semantic cueing, making it highly sensitive to early memory impairment, particularly in Alzheimer's disease (Grober et al, 2010). Spanish-language versions have been validated across several countries. In Spain, Bonete-López et al. (2020) tested a recognition adaptation in older adults (M age = 65.7, M education = 11.4 years), showing excellent internal consistency, ceiling-level recognition, and no significant sex or demographic effects. In Argentina, Labos et al. (2008) validated the test in 239 adults (M age = 56.4), demonstrating age-related declines from age 60 and significant effects of education on recall, though semantic cues benefitted all groups. The Spanish Multicenter Normative Studies, NEURONORMA project (Peña-Casanova et al, 2009) provided norms for over 600 Spanish participants aged 50–94, confirming robust age and education effects but minimal sex differences, with recall dropping up to 11% in those with lower schooling. Finally, the Coyoacán study in Mexico City (Mokri et al, 2013) provided culturally adapted norms (e.g., replacing the word for "flower" with "amapola") for over 1,000 adults aged 70+, showing that education strongly enhanced recall while age, especially above 80, was associated with a marked decline; recognition again showed ceiling effects.

Strengths and Limitations: The FCSRT's cross-cultural adaptations and large normative datasets make it a valuable benchmark for Spanish-speaking populations, particularly in detecting early AD-related memory changes. Its structured cueing improves sensitivity to encoding versus retrieval deficits, strengthening clinical utility. However, strong effects of age and education limit comparability across populations, and recognition scores often reach ceiling levels, reducing discriminative power in well-educated or younger groups.

CERAD Word List

The CERAD Word List Memory Task is structured in three stages: learning, delayed recall, and recognition. In the learning phase, participants study 10 words, each displayed on a card for two seconds, across three trials, with the total learning score based on the number of words recalled correctly across trials (maximum = 30). After a 10-minute interval, they complete a free recall of the 10 words (maximum = 10). In the recognition phase, participants are presented with 20 words, including the 10 targets and 10 distractors, and must identify the previously studied items. Normative data for the Spanish version are detailed on Torres et al. (2021).

Strengths and Limitations: The CERAD Word List Memory Task is simple, reliable, and clinically useful for distinguishing memory processes such as encoding, storage, and retrieval. Its brevity makes it easy to administer, but the short 10-word list may limit sensitivity in highly educated individuals, and cultural or linguistic adaptations can affect comparability across populations.

The Loewenstein-Acevedo Scales for Semantic Interference and Learning

A cognitive challenge test (CCT) is designed to detect early cognitive vulnerabilities tied to specific disease processes and brain biomarkers. The Loewenstein-Acevedo Scales for Semantic Interference and Learning (LASSI-L), developed simultaneously in English and Spanish, is one such test that measures recovery from proactive semantic interference (PSI), failure to recover from PSI (frPSI), and semantic intrusion errors-processes shown to be highly sensitive to early Alzheimer disease-related changes (Curiel Cid et al, 2020; Crocco et al, 2018; Loewenstein et al, 2016). Validation studies have confirmed its strong psychometric properties: excellent test-retest reliability across subscales (e.g., Free Recall r = 0.55; Cued Recall r = 0.70), robust convergent validity with other memory measures such as the Fuld Object Memory Evaluation and the Semantic Interference Test, and discriminant validity in distinguishing amnestic MCI from normal cognition with sensitivity of 87.9% and specificity of 91.5% (Crocco et al, 2014; Curiel et al, 2018). U.S. norms were derived from 224 cognitively healthy adults aged 60–95, including English speakers, and

72 Spanish speakers stratified by age. Spanish-speaking participants reflected important generational differences in education, with older adults averaging 11.9 years versus 15 years in younger groups, highlighting the role of educational access in test performance.

> **Strengths and Limitations:** The LASSI-L's greatest strength lies in its design, targeting AD-specific memory processes and developed natively in Spanish as well as English, making it culturally and linguistically relevant. It has shown strong associations with AD biomarkers, and the availability of a digitized version increases accessibility and standardization. Its normative base is also more demographically inclusive than many traditional tests, capturing education-related disparities in older cohorts. However, its limitations include reliance on relatively modest sample sizes, particularly among Spanish speakers, and limited longitudinal data on predictive validity, leaving questions about how well it tracks disease progression over time.

The Spanish Versions of the Face-Name Associative Memory Exam (S-FNAME and LAS-FNAME)

The Face-Name Associative Memory Exam (FNAME) is a cross-modal associative learning test developed to detect subtle episodic memory deficits, particularly in preclinical Alzheimer's disease. The Spanish FNAME was adapted from the original English version and validated in Spain (Alegret et al, 2020; Alegret et al, 2015). The test requires learning and recalling 16 face-name and 16 face-occupation pairs with both immediate and delayed recall phases. Initial validation in a small memory clinic sample showed that education, age, and sex significantly influenced performance. These findings were later reinforced by larger community-based studies, such as the Barcelona Brain Health Initiative, where regression analyses again confirmed the impact of demographic variables, particularly age, gender, and education, on S-FNAME outcomes (Alviarez-Schulze et al, 2022). Factor analyses further confirmed that S-FNAME captures distinct cognitive processes, face-name and face-occupation associations, highlighting the test's ability to isolate specific aspects of associative memory; this is a valuable, subtle change that may precede prodromal clinical manifestations of AD.

The Latin American Spanish version of the FNAME (LAS-FNAME), adapted in Colombia with culturally and linguistically appropriate names, was validated in 59 cognitively normal adults (71% female) aged 27–82 years (M = 50.31, SD = 15.32) with 2–17 years of education (M = 9.02, SD = 4.11). Findings demonstrated strong internal consistency, solid convergent validity with other episodic memory measures, reliable test–retest performance, and meaningful associations with AD-related biomarkers, including amyloid and tau pathology (Vila-Castelar, Papp et al, 2020; Vila-Castelar, Munoz et al, 2020).

Strengths and Limitations: The FNAME and it's Spanish adaptations S-FNAME and LAS-FNAME, provide a sensitive measure of associative and episodic memory, with demonstrated internal consistency, convergent validity with established memory tests, and even associations with AD-related biomarkers, underscoring their clinical and research utility. Strengths include careful cultural and linguistic adaptations, rigorous psychometric validation, and evidence that the test captures subtle memory changes relevant to preclinical Alzheimer's disease. However, limitations arise from demographic influences, as performance is strongly affected by education, age, and sex, which may limit comparability across populations with diverse backgrounds. Normative samples have also been relatively small and region-specific (e.g., Catalonia and Colombia), raising concerns about generalizability to broader Spanish-speaking or bilingual populations. Additionally, the reliance on visual processing could disadvantage individuals with visual impairments, potentially confounding results.

VISUAL MEMORY

Brief Visuospatial Memory Test—Revised

The Brief Visuospatial Memory Test (BVMT) (Benedict, 1995) was developed to assess immediate and delayed visual memory. The revised version (BVMT-R) (Benedict, 1996) expanded the test by adding a learning component with three 10-second trials, as well as a recognition task to reduce reliance on graphomotor skills. In the NP-NUMBRS project, administration and scoring followed the original English protocol, awarding one point each for correct location and correct construction.

Normative data were collected from 254 Spanish-speaking adults living in the U.S.-Mexico border regions of California and Arizona across two cohorts (see page 7 for more details on the NP-NUMBRS project). For the BVMT-R, participants were randomly assigned to Form 1 (n = 138) or Form 2 (n = 64). Analyses showed that English-speaking White norms overestimated impairment in this sample, while Black/African American norms from the San Diego region yielded impairment rates closer to those observed in the Spanish-speaking cohort. This suggests that differences in impairment rates are not solely attributable to language.

> **Strengths and Limitations:** The NP-NUMBRS project offers several strengths, including regression-based norms derived from relatively small samples, co-normed tests, and demonstrated sensitivity in detecting HIV-associated neurocognitive impairment. However, limitations include uneven site recruitment (Arizona versus California), restricted age coverage (excluding children and older adults), reliance on self-reported education that may not capture literacy or education quality, and potential cohort effects given that data were collected more than a decade ago.

Batería Neuropsicológica en Español—Memoria Visual

The Batería Neuropsicológica en Español (BNE) Visual Memory Test, adapted from Heaton et al. (1991) evaluates visual learning, retrieval, and retention of geometric shapes using three cards from the original 1945 Wechsler Memory Scale. Each card is shown for 10 seconds, with examinees reproducing the figures across up to five learning trials unless 15 details are recalled earlier. A one-hour incidental delay precedes recall and recognition trials.

Artiola Fortuny et al. (1998) developed norms from 390 participants, including 205 from Madrid and 185 from the U.S.-Mexico border (Nogales, Agua Prieta, and Tucson). Full inclusion and exclusion criteria are described in (Artiola i Fortuny, Heaton, and Hermosillo, 1998) and (Artiola i Fortuny, 1996). The study also excluded individuals with a high level of education who reported difficulties with reading, writing, or mathematics in childhood. Regression-based analyses adjusted for age and education, with validation achieved by splitting the sample. Independent studies of sensitivity and specificity, however, are lacking.

Strengths and Limitations: Strengths include regression-based norms, smaller required sample sizes, and coverage of both Spanish and U.S. Latino groups. Limitations involve limited geographic generalizability, lack of rural representation, and the lengthy one-hour delay, which can be burdensome in practice.

NEUROPSI—Attention and Memory

Includes a design to test non-verbal memory. See pages 20–21 (Ostrosky-Solis et al, 2007) for a description of the norms.

Rey-Osterrieth Complex Figure

The norms for the recall of the Rey-Osterrieth Complex Figure (ROCF) and the Benson Complex Figure are described in the next section.

VISUOSPATIAL CONSTRUCTIONAL ABILITIES

Rey–Osterrieth Complex Figure

The copy and immediate recall of the Rey-Osterrieth Complex Figure (ROCF), first designed by (Rey, 1941) and standardized by (Osterrieth, 1944a), is widely used to assess visual perception and visuospatial constructional ability, and immediate nonverbal memory (Corwin, 1993). Beyond these core functions, the ROCF also provides information about organizational strategies, problem-solving, planning, attention, concentration, and fine motor coordination.

Several large-scale normative projects have examined the ROCF in Spanish-speaking groups. (Rivera, Perrin, Weiler et al, 2015) collected data from 3,968 healthy adults across 10 Latin American countries and Puerto Rico, using stringent inclusion criteria. Due to limited sample sizes within some education categories, years of education were dichotomized (1–12 versus >12). As part of a large-scale normative study of Spanish-speaking adults in the U.S., including 245 individuals, 18–80 years old, from California, Connecticut, Florida, Indiana, New Jersey, Oregon, Virginia, Wisconsin, (Morel Valdes et al, 2024) investigated how age, education, language proficiency, and time in the U.S. influence performance on the ROCF. Using Bayesian regression analyses, the authors examined the effects of bilingualism, acculturation, and demographic variables on test outcomes. They found that ROCF performance was significantly influenced by age, education, language proficiency, and duration of residence in the U.S. Older adults with stronger Spanish proficiency or balanced bilingualism made more errors in copy, recall, and memory decay tasks, whereas higher English proficiency was associated with better overall performance. Education improved performance and reduced memory decay, and its interaction with time in the U.S. showed that extended residency worsened outcomes for less educated participants but benefited those with higher education.

Palomo et al. (2013) provided Spanish norms for 332 community-dwelling adults over age 49, administering copy, a three-minute immediate recall, a delayed recall after 30 minutes, and a recognition task following the scoring guidelines in Meyers (1995). Unlike other studies, they permitted participants with stable medical or psychiatric histories. Age was stratified into narrow three-year bands, education into seven levels, and analyses used overlapping intervals and regression-based adjustments for age and education. Although this approach increased ecological validity, generalizability was limited by non-epidemiologic sampling and an asymmetrical distribution skewed toward older adults. The NEURONORMA norms were subsequently validated in clinical populations, including MCI, AD, and multiple sclerosis.

Torres et al. (2021) developed norms from 2,673 Colombian participants in the API Registry. For adults over age 40, education was dichotomized into low versus high attainment due to small cell sizes. Additional combined norms were provided for participants over age 60. While the large sample and detailed stratification were strengths, limitations included a young skew, regional recruitment confined to Antioquia, and variability in educational quality between rural and urban participants.

Finally, Ostrosky-Solis et al. (2007) incorporated the ROCF copy and 20-minute delay into the Neuropsi Atención y Memoria battery. This dataset provided broad age and education coverage across Spanish-speaking countries and demonstrated clinical reliability. However, the use of wide educational bands (10–22 years) may reduce interpretability for individuals at the extremes of schooling.

Strengths and Limitations: Normative studies of the ROCF in Spanish-speaking populations demonstrate several strengths, including large sample sizes, broad geographic representation, and regression-based adjustments for demographic variables such as age and education. Projects like Rivera et al. (2015) and Torres et al. (2021) contribute valuable data from Latin America, while Palomo et al. (2013) and Ostrosky-Solis et al. (2007) provide detailed stratification and validation across clinical populations. These efforts enhance the clinical utility of the ROCF and support its use in diverse contexts. However, important limitations remain: many studies relied on convenience sampling rather than epidemiological recruitment, educational bands were often collapsed or overly broad, and some samples were skewed toward particular age groups or geographic regions. Given the strong influence of education on performance, these methodological issues reduce the generalizability of norms and highlight the need for culturally sensitive, demographically balanced reference data.

The NEUROPSI Semi-Complex Figure Test

Ostrosky-Solis et al. (1998) introduced the Semi-Complex Figure as an alternative to the ROCF for individuals with fewer than four years of education. Designed as a simplified copy-and-recall task, it retains the structure of the ROCF but with more discrete and less intricate elements. The scoring system is reduced to a maximum of 12 points, compared to 36 for the ROCF (Ostrosky-Solis, Ardila, and Rosselli, 1999). Unlike the ROCF, which typically includes a fixed delay, the Semi-Complex Figure was incorporated into the NEUROPSI Breve, a brief neuropsychological battery standardized for administration in 25–30 minutes.

Strengths and Limitations: The NEUROPSI Breve, including the Semi-Complex Figure, offers important advantages such as applicability across a wide age and education range, validation in multiple clinical groups (e.g., TBI in Colombia), and even adaptation for phone-based administration. It demonstrates good test–retest reliability and efficient administration time. However, its limitations include the use of broad demographic bands and normative data drawn exclusively from Mexico, which restricts the generalizability of its norms to other Latino populations.

Benson Figure Test

The Benson Figure Test (BFT) includes copy, immediate recall, and delayed recall conditions and was developed by Frank Benson as a simplified adaptation of the CFT (Kramer et al, 2003). Like the RCFT, it assesses visuoconstructional and visual memory abilities, but its design reduces executive and motor demands. The BFT is incorporated into Version 3.0 of the National Alzheimer's Coordinating Center Uniform Data Set Neuropsychological Battery (UDS3-NB) and has been validated in a large cohort of 3,602 cognitively normal adults over age 60 (Weintraub et al, 2018a). More recently, Marquine et al. (2023) published UDSNB 3.0 norms, including the BFT, in a Hispanic/Latino sample (see the first paragraph on page 8 for the sample details).

Strengths and Limitations: A key strength of the BFT is its reduced complexity, which makes it accessible for older adults and clinical populations where executive or motor demands may confound performance. However, limitations include restricted generalizability, as norms were drawn from ADRC-based recruitment with smaller sample sizes compared to other UDS3-NB studies. The Hispanic/Latino sample further lacked a detailed evaluation of culturally relevant factors such as acculturation, literacy, and education quality, while language use was self-reported and assessed only in a subset. Differences in bilingualism were observed but not fully analyzed, limiting interpretability.

Block Design (WAIS)

The Block Design subtest of the WAIS assesses visuomotor construction by requiring examinees to arrange four to nine mono-colored and bicolored blocks to replicate increasingly complex patterns.

Scott et al. (2021) developed norms for the WAIS-R Block Design, as part of the (NP-NUMBRS) project, including 254 Spanish-speaking adults recruited in the U.S.-Mexico border regions of Tucson, Arizona, and San Diego, California (see more details on page 7).

Strengths and Limitations: The use of regression-based, co-normed measures strengthens the NP-NUMBRS battery, improving sensitivity for Spanish-speaking adults and demonstrating validity in detecting HIV-associated impairment. However, norms are limited by recruitment from the U.S.-Mexico border region, exclusion of younger and older age groups, and reliance on convenience samples, which may restrict generalizability.

Judgment of Line Orientation

The Judgment of Line Orientation (JLO) was first developed by Benton et al. (1975) to assess visuospatial perception and orientation. The task requires examinees to judge angular relationships by visually matching two angled line pairs to line segments arranged as radii within a semicircle.

Normative data for Spanish speakers were later provided by (Pena-Casanova, Quintana-Aparicio et al, 2009) through the NEURONORMA Project (see pages 9–10 for project details). The main findings were that education had the strongest influence on performance, explaining 18% of the variance, while age accounted for only 3%. Sex also had a notable effect, explaining 5% of raw score variance and 8% after age adjustment, supporting the need for sex-based corrections. After adjusting for age, education continued to explain up to 14% of score variance, leading researchers to include education and sex adjustments in the final normative model. Correction tables were created to allow clinicians to adjust JLO scores for age, education, and sex using standardized NEURONORMA scaled scores.

Strengths and Limitations: The JLO is a widely used measure of visuospatial perception that shows strong construct validity and sensitivity to right parietal lobe dysfunction, with minimal language demands, making it suitable for diverse clinical populations. Its strengths include well-established clinical utility and broad applicability, but performance can be influenced by factors such as age, education, visual acuity, and motor abilities. These influences, along with potential cultural and educational differences, highlight the importance of using appropriate normative data when interpreting results.

Consortium to Establish a Registry for Alzheimer's Disease Constructional Praxis

The Consortium to Establish a Registry for Alzheimer's Disease (CERAD) Constructional Praxis evaluates visuoconstruction and memory through copy and delayed recall of four geometric figures, scored out of 11 points (Aguirre-Acevedo, 2007). Norms from Torres et al. (2021) based on the Colombian API Registry, provided a very large sample with broad age (18–86) and education (1–25 years) ranges, extending previous normative efforts and strengthening its applicability. See description of this study on page 18.

Strengths and Limitations: A key strength of this study is its unusually large sample size for a normative dataset, which increases reliability, along with the inclusion of wide age and education ranges. However, limitations include a skewed age distribution with many participants under age 30, the dichotomization of education levels for older adults, and restriction to Colombia, which limits generalizability.

Visual Object and Space Perception Battery

The Visual Object and Space Perception Battery (VOSP), developed by Warrington and James (1991) consists of eight tasks designed to assess object and space perception while ensuring that basic visual-sensory deficits do not confound performance (Strauss, Sherman, and Spreen, 2006). It was originally created to identify selective impairments associated with right-hemispheric brain damage.

Normative data for Spanish-speaking populations were established by Calvo et al. (2013) as part of the NEURONORMA Project (see pages 9–10 for project details). Their findings indicated that education had minimal influence on performance across all VOSP subtests, a result attributed to the absence of participants with fewer than eight years of education. Similarly, age showed no significant effect on performance, which the authors explained by the relatively young age range of the sample compared with previous studies. Consistent with earlier research, gender was not associated with differences in performance. The authors developed correction tables that allow clinicians to adjust scores for age and education using standardized NEURONORMA scaled scores, providing a reliable reference for the interpretation of VOSP results in Spanish-speaking individuals.

Strengths and Limitations: The VOSP battery is used to assess for right hemisphere dysfunction and, similar to other visual measures, benefits from minimal language demands. This makes it suitable for diverse populations. Its strengths include its wide use across a variety of neurodegenerative diseases, including posterior cortical atrophy, Lewy body dementia, Huntington's, and Parkinson's plus syndromes (Calvo et al, 2013). The aforementioned inconsistency of minimal to no influence of education and age, respectively, highlights the need for further exploration in normative studies, inclusive of older adults and greater educational variability (i.e., participants with education less than eight years).

MOTOR SKILLS

Grooved Pegboard Test & Finger Tapping Test

The Grooved Pegboard Test, developed in 1963 (Klove, 1963) and distributed by the Lafayette Instrument Company, measures fine motor speed and hand-eye coordination, requiring sensory-motor integration and higher-order motor processing. The Finger Tapping Test assesses gross motor speed, with roots in early 20th-century tapping experiments (Wells, 1909) and long-standing use in neuropsychological assessment (Reitan and Wolfson, 1985b; Kreutzer, DeLuca, and Caplan, 2018).

Heaton et al. (2021) provided normative data by administering both tests to 254 Spanish-speaking adults in the U.S.-Mexico border region (Arizona and California) across two cohorts: 183 participants recruited between 1998–2000 in Tucson, Texas, and San Diego, California, and 71 healthy controls from a 2006–2009 study of HIV outcomes in San Diego. These samples were combined to strengthen the normative dataset. A detailed description of the sample and procedures is presented under NP-NUMBRS on page 7.

> **Strengths and Limitations:** Strengths include regression-based norms, which enhance sensitivity for detecting impairment while reducing sample size requirements. However, the normative base is geographically limited to the U.S.-Mexico border region, which may constrain broader generalizability.

DEMENTIA STAGING SCALES

The Clinical Dementia Rating

The Clinical Dementia Rating (CDR) and its adaptations have been evaluated across Latino/Hispanic populations with attention to linguistic, cultural, and psychometric considerations. The Clinical Dementia Rating Dementia Staging Instrument (CDR-FTLD NACC) (UDSv3) quantifies dementia severity across six domains:

- Memory
- Orientation
- Judgment/Problem Solving
- Community Affairs
- Home/Hobbies
- Personal Care

Marquine et al. (2023) developed UDS3-NB norms (not CDR validation) for 437 Latino/Hispanic adults (ages 50–94) recruited from 33 National Institutes of Aging (NIA)-sponsored Alzheimer's Disease Research Centers (ADRCs), primarily before March 2020. Participants self-identified as Hispanic/Latino, were English- or Spanish-speaking, and were cognitively normal (CDR = 0). Spanish speakers were older and less educated, but sex distribution did not differ; nearly half were of Mexican descent.

The modified CDR (mCDR) was evaluated in Hispanic older adults with MCI, demonstrating moderate-to-good inter-rater reliability ($\beta \approx .72–73$) and strong convergent validity with the ADCS-MCI-ADL, which itself showed comparable reliability ($\beta = .71$) and remained consistent after controlling for language ($\beta = .72, p < .001$) (Mendoza, 2023).

Among Mexican Americans, Julayanont and DeToledo (2022) established CDR-SB cutoff ranges (0 = normal, 0.5–4 = MCI/very mild dementia, 4.5–8 = mild, 8.5–13 = moderate, 13.5–18 = severe). In 1,073 participants, the CDR-SB demonstrated high diagnostic accuracy, with thresholds valid even among those with <6 years of education, supporting its cross-educational utility.

Finally, linguistic adaptation has been addressed. The CDR was culturally tailored by Oquendo-Jimenez et al. (2010) for Puerto Rican Spanish; twenty-five semantic and four content modifications (e.g., everyday vocabulary and culturally relevant examples) were recommended, while preserving the scoring structure. However, no psychometric validation was conducted, highlighting the need for subsequent reliability and validity testing.

Strengths and Limitations: The CDR and its adaptations have proven useful for Hispanic/Latino populations, offering a structured assessment of cognitive and functional abilities with evidence of reliability, validity, and diagnostic accuracy. Cultural adaptations, such as the Puerto Rican Spanish version, have preserved conceptual equivalence (Oquendo-Jimenez et al, 2010). Nonetheless, limitations remain, including inconsistent diagnostic reporting, insufficient psychometric validation of some adaptations, and limited evaluation of the CDR in specific Latino subgroups (Marquine et al, 2023), underscoring the need for further culturally sensitive validation.

DIGITAL NEUROPSYCHOLOGICAL MEASURES

LASSI_L Digitized Version

The LASSI-L and its digital version, the LASSI-D, provide culturally and linguistically inclusive tools for assessing semantic interference, with both English and Spanish versions developed from inception. The LASSI-D modernizes the original paper-and-pencil format through cloud-based, voice-recognition software, enabling remote, standardized administration on computers, tablets, or smartphones in only 10–12 minutes.

Validation studies demonstrate that the LASSI-D preserves the psychometric strengths of the LASSI-L while enhancing efficiency and diagnostic sensitivity to early cognitive decline (Harvey et al, 2025). In community-based research involving 112 English- or Spanish-speaking adults over age 59, the LASSI-D demonstrated strong discriminative ability, reliably distinguishing cognitively unimpaired individuals from those with MCI without evidence of ceiling or floor effects. The sample reflected varied educational attainment, with 12% of LASSI-D participants having less than a high school education, 20% completing high school, 27% reporting some college, 22% being college graduates, and 18% holding advanced degrees. Importantly, the majority of participants identified as Hispanic/Latino, underscoring the measure's applicability across culturally and linguistically diverse populations (Curiel Cid et al, 2021; Curiel Cid et al, 2024). Normative data reflect demographic diversity: in one study conducted in Florida, 75% of the LASSI-D sample identified as Hispanic, and 45% were Spanish-speaking, with education ranging from less than high school to advanced degrees, demonstrating feasibility across backgrounds.

Extensive validation work links LASSI performance to biological markers of AD pathology. Deficits measured by the LASSI-L correlate with medial temporal lobe and precuneus volume loss (Loewenstein et al, 2017), while other studies confirm associations with amyloid burden and plasma Aβ42/40 (Curiel Cid et al, 2024), phosphorylated tau (p-tau181, p-tau217) (Curiel, 2013), and MRI indices of neurodegeneration (Loewenstein et al, 2017). These findings underscore the measure's utility for detecting preclinical and prodromal AD, where traditional tests often lack sensitivity.

Strengths and Limitations: The LASSI-D shows several strengths as a culturally inclusive tool for early detection of cognitive decline. Developed in English and Spanish, it uses cloud-based, voice-recognition software for efficient (10–12 minutes), standardized remote administration. Studies confirm it maintains the strong psychometric properties of the LASSI-L, with improved sensitivity to preclinical and prodromal AD, reliably differentiating unimpaired adults from those with MCI without ceiling or floor effects. Normative data from diverse, predominantly Hispanic/Latino samples with varied education further support its feasibility, while correlations with biomarkers of neurodegeneration strengthen its validity. Limitations include limited longitudinal data, small samples, the underrepresentation of Hispanic subgroups, and potential barriers related to technology access and digital literacy.

NIH Toolbox Cognition Battery

The NIH Toolbox Cognition Battery (NIHTB-CB) is a 30-minute computerized assessment of six cognitive domains through seven measures, including five tests of fluid abilities (problem-solving, reasoning, memory) and two tests of crystallized abilities (knowledge, language skills) (Casaletto et al, 2015). The Spanish version was developed through a rigorous translation and adaptation process using the FACIT methodology, including forward- and back-translation, expert review, and quality assurance steps (Beaumont et al, 2013; Casaletto et al, 2015; Casaletto et al, 2016). Psychometric validation supported the construct distinction between fluid and crystallized cognition, with item response theory analyses confirming that Spanish-language items were equivalent to the English versions. Convergent and divergent validity were established through strong correlations with traditional neuropsychological measures (e.g., the Rey Auditory Verbal Learning Test [RAVLT] and the Dimensional Change Card Sort Test [DCCS]) and weak correlations with unrelated domains, confirming test specificity (Casaletto et al, 2015).

To strengthen its clinical utility, demographically corrected normative data were developed for 408 Spanish-speaking neurologically healthy adults (ages 18–85), adjusting scores for age, education, and sex (Casaletto et al, 2016). The sample, primarily Hispanic/Latino White (77%), had a mean age of 44.1 years and a mean education of 10.7 years, with most (94%) reporting Spanish as their first language. While adjustments reduced group differences, performance was still influenced by sociocultural factors such as birthplace, bilingualism, and socioeconomic status. Importantly, 40.4% of participants scored at or below the 16th percentile on at least one fluid ability measure, highlighting the need for stratified base rates to contextualize performance across diverse Spanish-speaking populations.

Strengths and Limitations: The NIHTB-CB is a psychometrically robust, culturally adaptable tool with carefully developed norms for Spanish speakers, making it valuable for cross-linguistic and cross-cultural assessment. However, while it provides broad coverage of cognitive domains, it may lack diagnostic specificity for subtle impairments characteristic of AD/ADRD.

VALIDITY OF TEST PERFORMANCE AND SYMPTOM VALIDITY

The inclusion of both performance and symptom validity measures in neuropsychological assessment is essential to supporting the credible interpretation of test results. These measures provide empirical evidence regarding the examinee's level of effort and the authenticity of reported symptoms, thereby determining whether the obtained data can be interpreted with confidence. In the absence of demonstrated validity, the accuracy and clinical utility of the entire evaluation may be substantially compromised, increasing the risk of misinterpretation or diagnostic error.

Test of Memory Malingering

The Test of Memory Malingering (TOMM) (Tombaugh, 1999) is a performance validity measure widely used in neuropsychological evaluations to detect exaggerated or fabricated memory complaints for secondary gain. The task involves presenting 50 pictures, followed by an immediate yes/no recognition trial with corrective feedback.

Rivera et al. (2015) developed Spanish-language norms using a large sample of 2,266 healthy adults from Argentina, Bolivia, Chile, Mexico, Paraguay, Peru, and Puerto Rico. Participants were administered the TOMM as part of a broader neuropsychological battery, though details of the translation and adaptation process were not specified. A standardized five-step statistical procedure was used to generate norms. Inclusion criteria required participants to be 18–95 years old, born and residing in the country of testing, native Spanish speakers, literate with at least one year of formal education, and meeting clinical cutoffs (MMSE ≥ 23; PHQ-9 ≤ 4; Barthel Index ≥ 90). Individuals with neurological or psychiatric conditions, substance abuse history, systemic or metabolic illnesses associated with cognitive impairment, severe sensory deficits, or use of medications likely to impact cognition were excluded.

Ramos Usuga et al. (2024) established U.S. normative data for the Spanish version of the Test of Memory Malingering-2 (TOMM2) among Hispanic/Spanish-speaking adults. Data were collected from 188 participants across nine sites:

- California: n = 42
- Connecticut: n = 33
- Florida: n = 54
- Indiana: n = 9
- New Jersey: n = 27
- Oregon: n = 12
- Virginia: n = 36
- Wisconsin: n = 40
- Total: N = 245; ages 18–80

Data were collected using iPads provided by Multi-Health Systems Inc. (MHS) with a prerelease digital TOMM2 containing newly drawn, modified, and replaced images. The TOMM2 represents the first revision of the original TOMM, designed to improve cross-cultural fairness and universal accessibility. Following the Standards for Educational and Psychological Testing, MHS engaged a diverse expert panel to evaluate new items for cultural sensitivity and collaborated with academic researchers to validate the materials in varied, cognitively healthy samples. Results showed high average scores and better performance than the English-speaking sample, providing the first culturally appropriate normative data for U.S. Spanish speakers.

Arango-Lasprilla et al. (2024) examined the TOMM2's validity in a Spanish sample of 200 cognitively healthy adults aged 18–86 years (M = 46.18, SD = 18.27), 65% of whom were female. Participants had an average of 13.61 years of education (SD = 4.04; range = 3–23). All participants scored within passing ranges using English-language cutoffs, with only one false classification under a stricter criterion (<40 on Trial 1). Spanish adults achieved perfect scores on Trial 1 at over twice the rate of English-speaking individuals, and nearly all items met performance validity standards, confirming high specificity. Age was linked to slightly lower scores and education to marginally higher scores, with no gender effects. These results support the TOMM2's strong validity, reliability, and cross-cultural generalizability for Spanish-speaking adults in Spain.

Strengths and Limitations: The TOMM and its updated version, the TOMM2, demonstrate strong validity as measures of performance validity. The TOMM2 introduces important improvements, including a digital format and culturally reviewed items designed to enhance fairness and accessibility. The development of Spanish-language norms across several U.S. sites, along with an additional reference sample from Spain, provides the first culturally appropriate normative data for Spanish-speaking adults, strengthening its cross-cultural applicability and clinical value. Nevertheless, some limitations remain. Existing studies lack complete psychometric validation, and the samples have tended to overrepresent highly educated participants, which may reduce generalizability to individuals with lower education levels or from less represented Latino regions. Because the TOMM2 is not yet fully released, additional independent research will be essential to confirm its reliability and fairness across diverse Spanish-speaking populations.

Structured Interview of Malingered Symptomatology

The Structured Inventory of Malingered Symptomatology (SIMS) is a 75-item true/false screening measure designed to detect exaggerated or feigned psychiatric, cognitive, and neurological symptoms (Smith and Burger, 1997). A Spanish-language adaptation was first developed in Spain (Veiga, 2007), followed by broader validation studies in the U.S. (González Ordi, 2009). According to the SIMS manual (Widows, 2009), the adaptation relied on both simulation-based and known-groups methodologies and was tested across diverse populations.

Spanish norms were established from a total sample of 1,005 participants (M = 31.9 years, SD = 13.2; range = 17–71; 66.4% female), recruited from 16 sites, including hospitals, forensic centers, insurance companies, and rehabilitation facilities. The control group (n = 147; 70.7% female; M age = 23.6, SD = 8.8) was instructed to respond honestly, while the simulation group (n = 326; 75.5% female; M age = 22.5, SD = 6.9) was divided into subgroups instructed to simulate symptoms of psychosis, accidents, amnesia, intellectual disability, affective disorders, general malaise, or pain disorder. The clinical sample (n = 152; 50.7% female; Mage = 42.5, SD = 12.6) was drawn from mental health and rehabilitation settings.

Across the total sample, the Spanish SIMS showed excellent internal consistency (α = .94 overall; subscales ranging from .65–90). The psychosis, amnesia, and neurological impairment subscales demonstrated strong reliability (α > .80), while affective disorders and low intelligence subscales showed weaker reliability, warranting wider confidence intervals in interpretation. Factor analyses supported a five-subscale structure: psychosis, neurological impairment, amnestic disorders, low intelligence, and affective disorders. Although test-retest reliability was not directly assessed for the Spanish version, the Dutch adaptation reported a coefficient of .72 (Merckelbach, 2003). In a known-groups validation study (Ordi, 2010), the SIMS successfully differentiated probable malingerers (n = 34) from non-malingerers (n = 27) in a medicolegal context.

Strengths and Limitations: The Spanish adaptation of the SIMS has notable strengths, including strong overall reliability, broad validation across clinical, forensic, and medicolegal contexts, and evidence of discriminant validity for conditions such as chronic pain and affective disorders. Its large normative sample further supports its applicability in Spanish-speaking populations. However, the reliability of the affective and low intelligence subscales is weaker than recommended, and recent findings indicate that the low intelligence subscale shows little discriminatory power, highlighting the need for caution when interpreting results from specific subdomains.

Rey 15-Item Test

The Rey 15-Item Plus Recognition trial is a brief measure of visual memory and response validity in which participants view 15 related items for 10 seconds, reproduce them by drawing, and later complete a recognition trial with targets embedded among distractors (Boone et al, 2002). Normative data for Spanish-speaking populations remain limited, but Strutt et al. (2011) addressed this gap by validating the test in 130 cognitively intact, Spanish-speaking older adults (ages 50–69) living in Houston, Texas. Norms were stratified by education level (basic education: 6–12 years; college education: >13 years), with individuals having fewer than 6 years of schooling excluded. Participants were classified as primarily Spanish-speaking using both an expressive vocabulary measure in English and the Marin Acculturation Scale (Marín et al, 1987). Analyses showed that education and MMSE scores significantly influenced performance, with some low-education participants recalling fewer items than the original suggested cutoff (<9), raising concerns about misclassification. These findings demonstrated that cutoffs derived from primarily English-speaking White samples are not appropriate for Spanish-speaking populations.

Strengths and limitations: The Rey 15-Item Plus Recognition trial provides a brief, practical measure of visual memory and validity, with norms developed for Spanish-speaking older adults that account for education and language dominance. Its strengths include attention to acculturation and education effects, but limitations involve the narrow age range (50–69), exclusion of individuals with <6 years of education, reliance on self-reported cognitive health, and lack of a known-groups design, which restricts its broader applicability.

FUNCTIONAL SCALES

Incorporating functional assessment scales into the neuropsychological evaluation of older adults is essential, as cognitive test scores alone provide an incomplete picture of everyday functioning. Functional measures offer critical information about an individual's capacity to perform real-world activities, thereby enhancing diagnostic accuracy, informing treatment and care planning, and guiding determinations of functional independence.

Alzheimer's Disease Cooperative Study

The Alzheimer's Disease Cooperative Study (ADCS) developed several functional evaluation tools to assess activities of daily living (ADLs) across the spectrum of cognitive decline. These include the ADCS-ADL-MCI, designed to track functional evolution in individuals with mild cognitive impairment (MCI), and the ADCS-ADL-sev, tailored for patients with severe Alzheimer's disease (AD) (Potashman et al, 2023). Both scales are informant-based, relying on caregiver reports of patients' ability to perform daily tasks. The ADCS-ADL-sev contains 19 items spanning basic ADLs (feeding, bathing, grooming) and more complex instrumental ADLs (IADLs), such as managing finances and understanding time. Clinicians use these scales to detect subtle declines in complex IADLs while noting preserved basic functioning, thereby improving diagnostic accuracy and monitoring disease progression.

The ADCS-ADL, a broader 23-item scale, has been widely used in U.S. clinical trials and practice since its development (Galasko et al, 1997; Galasko et al, 2005). It evaluates both basic and instrumental ADLs, with scores ranging from 0 (total dependence) to 78 (full independence), based on caregiver reports of the patient's performance in the prior four weeks. Validation studies have shown its sensitivity in distinguishing MCI from early AD and in tracking functional decline over time, contributing to its widespread adoption in both research and clinical settings. However, normative data are currently available only for English-speaking populations, and while the ADCS reports that there is a Spanish translation, details about specific adaptations and norms remain unpublished.

A Spanish-language validation was conducted in Peru (Custodio et al, 2022), where 276 participants were classified into AD (n = 113), MCI (n = 68), and cognitively healthy controls (n = 95). While the study did not detail the translation/adaptation process, results indicated excellent test-retest reliability and satisfactory internal consistency. Some items (e.g., walking, reading, and hobbies) showed weaker correlations with total scores, and limitations included recruitment from a specialized center in Lima and non-random sampling, potentially reducing generalizability. Researchers also noted that the scale may be outdated due to technological and lifestyle changes accelerated by the COVID-19 pandemic. Despite these limitations, the Peruvian validation highlights the potential of the ADCS-ADL as a functional assessment tool for Spanish-speaking populations, addressing a gap in culturally adapted measures.

Strengths and Limitations: The ADCS-ADL scales offer several strengths, including strong validation in U.S. clinical and research settings, sensitivity to functional decline across the spectrum from MCI to severe AD, and informant-based reporting that captures both basic and instrumental daily activities. Their widespread adoption in clinical trials reflects their reliability, ability to track disease progression, and utility for care planning. However, limitations include the lack of publicly available normative data for non-English-speaking populations, limited cultural and linguistic adaptations, and evidence that some items may be outdated or less relevant given technological and lifestyle changes. Studies outside the U.S., such as the Peruvian validation, also note sampling constraints that may limit generalizability.

The Activities of Daily Living Questionnaire

Originally developed in English (Johnson et al, 2004), the Activities of Daily Living Questionnaire (ADLQ) was adapted into Spanish (Gleichgerrcht et al, 2009) through a study involving caregivers of 40 patients with various types of dementia recruited from the Institute of Cognitive Neurology (INECO) in Buenos Aires, Argentina. The adaptation process included two independent translations into Spanish followed by two back-translations into English, which were reviewed by the original author to ensure conceptual equivalence. The Spanish version maintained the original structure, consisting of six items on self-care, six on household care, four on employment and recreation, three on shopping and money, four on travel, and five on communication. After demonstrating strong internal consistency and concurrent validity, the ADLQ-SV was established as the Spanish adaptation.

A subsequent version, the Technology Activities of Daily Living Questionnaire (T-ADLQ) (Munoz-Neira et al, 2012), was developed in 2012 to assess functional abilities related to technology use. This version was validated using reports from 63 caregivers of dementia patients, 21 proxies of individuals with mild cognitive impairment, and 44 proxies of cognitively normal older adults. The T-ADLQ showed adequate validity and reliability, although the inclusion of technology-related items did not enhance the overall performance of the scale.

Strengths and Limitations: Small sample size in the initial validation of the questionnaire in Spanish, and only the presence of patients with bvFTD and Alzheimer's disease patients was assessed. However, the authors note that the strong internal consistency and validity are major considerations for the future use of this instrument. For the technology version, the use of technology did not improve the performance of the scale to measure functionality; however, it adds an important domain that needs to be taken into consideration for future generations.

The Functional Activity Questionnaire

The Functional Activity Questionnaire (FAQ) is a widely used measure of functional status in activities of daily living (Pfeffer et al, 1982). It consists of ten items rated on a scale from 0 (normal) to 3 (dependent) and is completed by a caregiver. A Spanish version, known as the "Cuestionario de Evaluación Funcional," was developed through Kaiser Permanente and has been incorporated into major dementia research programs such as the Alzheimer's Disease Neuroimaging Initiative (ADNI) and the National Alzheimer's Coordinating Center (NACC). Despite its extensive use, the NACC recently examined the FAQ's reliability and validity in a large cohort including both English and Spanish speakers (Gonzalez et al, 2022). The study evaluated 1,281 Spanish-speaking participants. Reliability was analyzed through internal consistency, test–retest assessments, and generalizability studies, while validity was examined through convergence with neurocognitive measures, classification accuracy across impairment stages, and confirmatory factor and item response theory analyses.

Strengths and Limitations: The FAQ is one of the most used questionnaires to measure functionality, with 10 simple items. However, there has not been a wide validation or reliability of this particular questionnaire in the Hispanic/Latino population, as well as Spanish speakers. Validation and reliability have proven to be adequate for its use in research and clinical settings after conducting these analyses in a large cohort of participants with extensive studies in both English and Spanish.

The Everyday Cognition

The Everyday Cognition (ECog) measures performance of activities of daily living in older adults with memory disorders, considering independence and autonomy (Farias et al, 2008). The validation for Spanish speakers was performed by Russo et al, 2018 in a cohort of older adults from the Argentina-ADNI study. The sample consisted of 15 clinically normal older adults, 28 mild cognitive impairment and 13 Alzheimer's disease patients. For this particular version of the ECog, 39 items were included to measure cognitive changes in the last 10-year period in six cognitive domains: memory, language, visuospatial and perceptive abilities, planning, organization, and divided attention. Response options include the following:

- 1 = better or no change compared to 10 years earlier
- 2 = questionable/occasionally worse
- 3 = consistently a little worse
- 4 = consistently much worse

An additional response of 0 is available for "I don't know." An ANOVA analysis was performed to observe variation between groups, with the addition of measuring both the Receiver operating characteristic (ROC) curve analysis and area under the curve (AUC) to discriminate power between the two groups. Diagnostic accuracy established the sensitivity and specificity of this test.

A Mexican version of this questionnaire (Aguilar-Navarro et al, 2023) was validated with a sample of 200 participants, older than 60, and their caregivers. The sample included 50 cognitively healthy participants, 50 with sickle cell disease, 50 with MCI, and 50 with dementia. The ECog version utilized in this study included the evaluation of six cognitive domains through 41 items, differing from the version of Russo et al. (2018). As described before, each item uses a Likert scale from 1 = better or no change to 4 = consistently much worse, with 0 as "I don't know." Higher cognitive impairment is indicated with higher scores in this scale (0–164 points). The authors examined group differences using ANOVA, and internal consistency was evaluated with Cronbach's alpha coefficient. Results showed this version to be a reliable and valid measure.

Strengths and Limitations: It has been validated across multiple studies, demonstrating consistent validity and reliability, showing strong accuracy in distinguishing cognitively impaired individuals from those who are cognitively healthy. In the Argentinian version, the authors acknowledged that their sample size was limited; however, the population was extensively examined by a diverse group of professionals. The authors also noted that the study used cross-sectional rather than longitudinal data, suggesting that longitudinal approaches may be more effective in demonstrating additional prognostic value.

PSYCHIATRIC INVENTORIES

Psychiatric inventories are a crucial component of neuropsychological assessment because they help clinicians understand the emotional, behavioral, and psychiatric factors that may influence cognitive functioning.

Beck Depression Inventory-II

The Beck Depression Inventory-II (BDI-II) is a 21-item self-report measure designed to assess the severity of depressive symptoms in individuals ≥13 years (Beck, Steer, and Brown, 1996).

The Spanish adaptations of the BDI-II have shown strong psychometric properties across diverse populations. In a community sample of 470 Spanish adults, Sanz et al. (2003) reported high internal consistency (α = 0.89) and a clear two-factor structure reflecting cognitive-affective and somatic-motivational dimensions. Normative data indicated slightly higher mean scores than the earlier BDI-IA, supporting an upward adjustment of cut-off points for depression severity.

In a medical sample of 122 Spanish-speaking hemodialysis patients, Penley et al. (2003) found excellent reliability (α = 0.92) and an adequate model fit (CFI = 0.76), suggesting the instrument's suitability in medically ill populations with varying levels of acculturation and socioeconomic status.

Among Puerto Rican older adults, Rodríguez-Gómez et al. (2006) identified four interpretable factors—somatic, cognitive-behavioral, biological, and negative attitudes—accounting for 52.83% of the variance, with strong reliability (α = 0.89). The mean BDI-II score was 7.90 (SD = 7.63), offering valuable normative data for elderly Spanish-speaking populations. Overall, the Spanish BDI-II demonstrates robust reliability, sound factorial validity, and solid normative foundations across community, clinical, and elderly groups.

Strengths and Limitations: The Spanish versions of the Beck Depression Inventory-II (BDI-II) demonstrate strong psychometric properties across diverse samples, showing high internal consistency (α ranging from 0.89–0.92) and stable factorial structures that capture both cognitive-affective and somatic aspects of depression. The availability of normative data from community, clinical, and elderly populations enhances its applicability and interpretive value across contexts. Its sensitivity to demographic and cultural factors further supports its utility in Spanish-speaking groups. However, some limitations include variations in factor structures across studies, which may reflect cultural or contextual influences, and limited evidence on its longitudinal validity or sensitivity to treatment effects. Additionally, most studies relied on specific regional samples, which may constrain generalization to other Spanish-speaking populations.

Beck Anxiety Inventory

The Beck Anxiety Inventory (BAI) is a 21-item self-report measure that assesses the severity of anxiety symptoms over the past week (Beck, Steer, and Brown, 1993). The Spanish adaptations of the BAI have shown strong psychometric properties across clinical and non-clinical samples. In a normative study with 1,467 participants from Madrid, including patients, community adults, and university students, the BAI demonstrated excellent internal consistency (α between .88 and .91) and good diagnostic validity, effectively distinguishing between individuals with and without anxiety disorders (AUC = .80). Independent centile tables were developed for each population and by gender, allowing for accurate interpretation of anxiety severity.

Further validation studies confirmed the measure's robustness. Magán et al. (2008) reported high reliability (α = .93) and a clear factorial structure with somatic and affective-cognitive components in a representative Spanish community sample. Sanz-Morejón et al. (2014) found similarly strong reliability (α = .91) and temporal stability (r = .84) in a clinical population of 918 patients, with two correlated dimensions explaining over 40% of variance. Overall, the Spanish BAI demonstrates excellent reliability, solid factorial validity, and comprehensive normative data that enhance its utility for both research and clinical assessment across Spanish-speaking populations.

Strengths and Limitations: The BAI demonstrates excellent reliability and validity across both clinical and community samples, with consistently high internal consistency (α ranging from .88–.93) and strong factorial and diagnostic validity. The availability of normative data for different populations and separate centile tables by gender enhances the accuracy of score interpretation and its clinical usefulness. Its stable two-factor structure, representing somatic and affective-cognitive symptoms, supports its conceptual clarity and applicability across diverse settings. However, some limitations include reliance on self-report data, which may be influenced by response bias, and variability in factor structures across studies, suggesting that cultural or contextual factors might affect symptom interpretation. Additionally, most validation studies have been cross-sectional, limiting conclusions about the measure's sensitivity to change over time.

Brief Symptom Inventory-18

The Brief Symptom Inventory-18 (BSI-18) is the most concise of Derogatis' instruments for assessing psychological distress. Andreu et al. (2008) validated the Spanish version in a clinical sample of 200 psychiatric outpatients in Madrid, ages 16–70 (M = 38.4), of whom 55% were women. The sample was clinically diverse, with the majority diagnosed with anxiety disorders (53.4%) or major depressive disorder (32%), while smaller proportions presented with adjustment, personality, eating, psychotic, or somatoform disorders. The BSI-18 was administered at baseline, retested in 103 participants after 15 days, and again in 31 patients after completion of psychological treatment to examine sensitivity to change. Internal consistency was satisfactory, with Cronbach's α values of .71 for anxiety, .88 for depression, and .89 for the total scale. Test-retest reliability was high, with the lowest correlation of .68 observed for the General Anxiety factor. Validity analyses conducted with 69 participants who also completed the BDI, BAI, and MMPI-2 demonstrated strong convergent and discriminant validity, with correlations between the BSI-18 total score and all measures exceeding $r = .74$ ($p < .001$).

> **Strengths and Limitations:** Overall, the Spanish BSI-18 demonstrated robust psychometric properties and sensitivity to therapeutic change, though its generalizability is constrained by the limited sample size, the underrepresentation of certain disorders, and the lack of non-clinical norms or deeper exploration of cultural influences on interpretation.

Generalized Anxiety Disorder-7

The Generalized Anxiety Disorder-7 (GAD-7) (Spitzer et al, 2006) is a brief, one-dimensional scale designed to measure symptoms of generalized anxiety disorder. In Spain, Garcia-Campayo et al. (2010) validated the instrument in a sample of 212 participants, including 106 patients with GAD and 106 controls, with an average age of 47.6 years and a predominance of women (73%). Diagnostic status was confirmed using DSM-IV-TR criteria and the Hamilton Anxiety Scale. The GAD-7 demonstrated excellent psychometric performance in this sample, with Cronbach's α of .94, a test-retest correlation of .84, and an intraclass correlation coefficient of .93. Criterion validity was confirmed by large group differences in total scores (M = 13.96 for GAD patients versus 3.54 for controls, $p < .001$), and the ROC curve yielded an AUC of .96, with a cutoff score of 10 providing strong sensitivity (86.8%) and specificity (93.4%). Additional evidence comes from Hispanic samples. Mills et al. (2014) studied 436 Mexican American adults divided into English- and Spanish-speaking groups, reporting excellent internal consistency (α = .91–.94) and strong correlations with perceived stress, depressive symptoms, and quality of life. Similarly, Pagán-Torres (2020) examined 302 Puerto Rican adults (74% female, mean age = 35.8) and found internal consistency ranging from α = .87–.92 and positive correlations with depression and PTSD measures.

Strengths and limitations: Collectively, these studies demonstrate the GAD-7's reliability, validity, and cultural adaptability across Spanish-speaking contexts, though limitations include regional focus, limited data on elderly populations, and uneven education levels that may affect broader generalizability.

Geriatric Depression Scale

The Geriatric Depression Scale (GDS) (Yesavage, 1986) is a widely used screening tool for depression in older adults, with several Spanish-language validations. Martínez de la Iglesia (2002) adapted the short version for Spain in a study of 249 elderly patients (M = 74.3, 68% women), most of whom had low or no formal education. Administered in primary care, the Spanish GDS demonstrated high internal consistency (α = .99) and diagnostic utility, with cutoffs between 4 and 7 balancing sensitivity and specificity across cognitively intact and impaired groups. Fernandez-San Martin et al. (2002) extended this work in 218 primary care patients in Madrid, confirming good reliability (α = .82) and applicability even among individuals with comorbid conditions or psychotropic use. In U.S. populations, Baker and Espino (1997) administered the GDS-15 to 41 Mexican American elders (M = 74) with depressive disorders, but the small sample yielded mixed accuracy in distinguishing MDD from other depression diagnoses and did not report reliability estimates. Broader validation was conducted by Bugallo-Carrera et al. (2023) in Galicia with 573 older adults (M = 70), finding stronger psychometric performance for the GDS-15 (α = .72, ROC = .76) than the GDS-5 (α = .50, ROC = .62). Lucas-Carrasco (2012) focused on 91 community-dwelling individuals with mild to moderate dementia (M = 79), reporting strong reliability for both GDS-15 (α = .81) and GDS-5 (α = .72), with significant correlations to clinician-rated depression and quality-of-life measures. Carrete et al. (2001) validated a telephone-administered version in 282 elderly Hispanics, showing equivalence with face-to-face administration and high reliability (α = .85–.88).

Strengths and Limitations: Spanish adaptations of the GDS show strong reliability and clinical utility across elderly populations, including those with low literacy, cognitive impairment, and dementia. Studies in Spain consistently report good internal consistency, sensitivity, and specificity, with the GDS-15 outperforming shorter forms like the GDS-5. Validation in dementia, telephone-administered formats, and among individuals with minimal education or psychotropic use underscores its flexibility and real-world applicability. However, most research is limited to Spain and select Hispanic groups, restricting generalizability. Small samples, underrepresentation of subgroups, lack of structured diagnostic interviews, and weaker performance of shorter versions further limit conclusions. Cultural and socioeconomic factors may also affect validity, and evidence in institutionalized or severely impaired patients remains sparse.

Geriatric Anxiety Inventory

Researchers examined the psychometric properties of the Spanish version of the Geriatric Anxiety Inventory (GAI) among 302 community-dwelling older adults in Spain (Marquez-Gonzalez et al, 2012). The participants had a mean age of 71.68 years (SD = 6.85) and averaged 11.3 years of formal education. The Spanish GAI demonstrated strong reliability with good internal consistency ($\alpha = 0.91$). Factor analysis revealed a three-factor structure comprising cognitive symptoms, arousal-related symptoms, and somatic symptoms, which explained 50.11% of the variance in responses. Criterion validity was established through significant associations between GAI scores and related measures, including depression, rumination, experiential avoidance, and emotion suppression. Demographic analyses showed that women scored higher than men on anxiety measures, while higher age and lower education levels were associated with greater anxiety symptoms.

Strengths and Limitations: The Spanish version of the GAI showed strong reliability and a clear three-factor structure capturing cognitive, arousal-related, and somatic symptoms. Its significant associations with related constructs support good criterion validity, and the relatively large community sample strengthens its applicability to non-clinical older adults. However, the exclusive focus on community-dwelling participants and the cross-sectional design limit conclusions about predictive validity and generalization to clinical or more diverse Spanish-speaking populations.

Symptom Checklist 90-R

The SCL-90-R (Derogatis, 1975) is a multidimensional measure of psychopathology symptoms. In Spain, De las Cuevas (1991) evaluated the Spanish version with a sample of 570 adults (ages 18–74, 52.5% female) without psychiatric symptoms. Adapted by González de Rivera (1989), the Spanish SCL-90-R produced factor structures broadly consistent with the original, with 84 of the 90 items showing strong correlations with intended symptom dimensions.

Strengths and Limitations: The findings indicate that the Spanish SCL-90 reproduces symptom dimensions similar to the original version, although six items showed weaker performance. However, the lack of detailed data on reliability, validity, and sensitivity prevents a full assessment of its diagnostic soundness, and the evidence remains limited to the Spanish population in which it was tested.

Patient Health Questionnaire-9

The PHQ-9 (Kroenke, Spitzer, and Williams, 2001) is a self-report measure of depressive symptoms. Rosario-Hernandez et al. (2023) evaluated its use in Puerto Rico across two studies involving 969 participants (55% women) divided into age groups from young to late adulthood, with an average of 15 years of education. The measure showed reliable response patterns and structural validity, with somatic items scoring slightly higher on average and all items showing consistent psychometric behavior, though item 9 (suicidality) was less stable. The PHQ-9 demonstrated validity for detecting depressive symptoms without major influence from demographic or social desirability factors. In a U.S. community study, Merz et al. (2011) administered the PHQ-9 to 479 Hispanic American women in San Diego (245 English-speaking and 234 Spanish-speaking), ages 18–80. Both groups demonstrated strong internal consistency (α = .84–.85) and equivalent one-factor structure, with 12.9% meeting clinical cutoff scores for depression. Mean scores did not significantly differ by language group, and measurement invariance was confirmed across English and Spanish versions. While item 9 loaded weakly on the factor, its clinical importance for suicide risk was underscored.

> **Strengths and Limitations:** Together, these studies demonstrate the PHQ-9's reliability, validity, and cross-language equivalence, although limitations include regional focus (Puerto Rico, Mexican-American women), limited inclusion of men or elderly adults, and the absence of diagnostic interviews in some samples.

State and Train Anxiety Inventory

The State and Train Anxiety Inventory (STAI) was first developed in Spanish in 1971 by Spielberger and colleagues using bilingual undergraduates from Texas and Puerto Rico. A short Spanish version was later created by Buela-Casal and Guillén-Riquelme (2017) using a non-probabilistic sample of 1,157 adults from Spain, divided into two random groups for discriminant and confirmatory factor analyses, along with a small clinical sample of 30 adults diagnosed with generalized anxiety disorder. Another reduced version, the STAIr, was developed by Fernández-Blázquez et al. (2015) in a sample of 489 older adults with a mean age of 74.34, also divided into development and validation groups. Using item response theory and a dichotomous Rasch model, the authors selected six items for the State scale and seven for the Trait scale, achieving high separation reliability and strong correlations with the original STAI.

Strengths and Weaknesses: Both short forms of the STAI offer clear strengths, particularly their brevity, strong model fit, and adequate psychometric properties, which make them useful for rapid assessment and for populations that benefit from simplified formats, such as older adults or individuals with cognitive changes. The STAIr also showed strong correlations with the full STAI, supporting the validity of its reduced item set. However, several limitations affect both measures. Each was developed using non-probabilistic samples from Spain, which restricts generalizability to Spanish-speaking populations in Latin America or the U.S., and the younger adult sample in the short-STAI may not reflect older clinical populations. The reduction in items for the STAIr likely weakened reliability, and limited information on educational variability leaves uncertainty about its suitability for individuals with lower literacy levels.

BEHAVIORAL INVENTORIES

Behavioral inventories are an essential component of neuropsychological assessment because they help evaluate how changes in the brain affect emotional, behavioral, and social functioning, areas that are often not fully captured by standard cognitive tests. These inventories provide a structured way to assess observable behaviors, personality changes, and psychological symptoms, all of which are critical for accurate diagnosis and treatment planning.

The Neuropsychiatric Inventory Questionnaire

The Neuropsychiatric Inventory Questionnaire (NPI-Q) is a brief derivative of the original Neuropsychiatric Inventory (NPI), the gold standard for assessing neuropsychiatric symptoms (NPS) in dementia and related disorders (Cummings et al, 1994). The original NPI measured 10 domains, later expanded to 12 with the addition of night-time disturbances and appetite/eating changes. The NPI-Q retains these domains while reducing administration time, making it particularly suitable for clinical and research contexts where brevity is essential. In addition to symptom frequency and severity, it captures associated caregiver distress.

Validation studies across Spanish-speaking populations confirm its strong psychometric properties. The Spanish version (Boada et al, 2002), developed through cross-validation with 120 Alzheimer's patients, demonstrated excellent test-retest reliability ($r = 0.89$ for total symptoms, $r = 0.90$ for distress) and robust convergent validity with the full NPI ($r = 0.879$ and $r = 0.92$, respectively). A Mexican study (Zepeda, 2008) involving 87 older adult dyads (mean age 79.4; 65.5% women; mean education 7.09 years; 10.3% illiterate) further confirmed its reliability ($\alpha = 0.778$; test-retest $r = 0.829$, ICC = 0.824) and validity, with significant correlations with MMSE ($r = 0.190$, $p = 0.001$), GDS ($r = 0.385$, $p = 0.0001$), and the NPI-D ($r = 0.887$, $p < 0.001$). The NPI-D itself showed excellent reliability (test-retest $r = 0.986$, ICC = 0.857, $\alpha = 0.779$) and strong links with caregiver burden ($r = 0.555$), while domain-specific analyses highlighted associations with sleep ($r = 0.731$), depression ($r = 0.402$), oral intake ($r = -0.335$), and psychosis ($r = 0.342$).

Additional evidence comes from a Chilean validation study (Musa et al, 2017) including 53 mild-to-moderate patients with AD (mean age 73.8; 41.5% women). Compared with the full NPI, the NPI-Q showed strong convergent validity for total symptoms ($r = 0.730$, $p < 0.01$) and distress ($r = 0.715$, $p < 0.01$), good internal consistency ($\alpha = 0.783$), and clear symptom prevalence patterns, with apathy (62.3%), depression (58.5%), and irritability (52.8%) most commonly. Symptom prevalence increased with disease severity, except for nighttime disturbances.

Beyond country-specific validations, measurement invariance was tested across 311 Hispanic and 10,863 non-Hispanic White outpatients, comparing the NPI-Q with the FAQ. Analyses supported configural and factorial invariance, and the NPI-Q demonstrated structural invariance with a four-factor model (hyperactivity, affect, psychosis, apathy/vegetative symptoms). However, scalar invariance was not achieved, meaning direct ethnic-group comparisons of severity levels are inappropriate, although within-group use is valid (Sayegh and Knight, 2014).

Strengths and Limitations: The NPI-Q consistently shows high reliability and convergent validity ($r \approx 0.88$–0.92) across Spanish-speaking populations, with broad applicability across varied educational and demographic contexts. Its brevity, coverage of 12 NPS domains, inclusion of caregiver distress, and clinically meaningful four-factor structure make it highly practical. Nevertheless, limitations include small sample sizes in some studies (e.g., Chile, $n = 53$), limited demographic reporting (e.g., Spain), and the absence of scalar invariance between Hispanic and non-Hispanic Whites, which restricts cross-group comparisons. As a screening tool, it cannot match the depth of the full NPI, and reliance on caregiver reports may introduce bias.

Social Behavior Observer Checklist

The Social Behavior Observer Checklist (SBOCL) is a brief tool for detecting subtle social behavior changes in older adults, distinguishing patients with conditions such as FTD and AD from cognitively healthy peers (Rankin et al, 2021). The final 14-item checklist is completed in 1–3 minutes, with examiners rating the severity of specific behaviors, such as insensitivity to privacy or embarrassment, on a four-point scale from "not at all" to "severely." This format allows a more nuanced assessment than binary checklists. The measure is available in Spanish; however, no published validation studies or normative data exist for Spanish-speaking populations, whether in the U.S. or abroad.

Strengths and Limitations: The SBOCL's brevity, structured four-point response scale, and targeted focus on social behaviors make it highly feasible in clinical settings, particularly for busy practitioners. Its availability in Spanish improves accessibility, and the observer-based format captures behaviors that may elude self-report. Yet major limitations restrict clinical interpretation: no normative data, no validation studies in Spanish-speaking groups, limited psychometric information overall, and the absence of established cutoffs or interpretive guidelines. In addition, reliance on trained raters raises the risk of bias and may limit feasibility in under-resourced settings.

Executive Interview

The Executive Interview (EXIT-25) is a structured screening tool for executive dysfunction that assesses domains such as perseveration, imitation, echopraxia, echolalia, intrusions, frontal release signs, spontaneity, disinhibition, and utilization behavior (Royall, Mahurin, and Gray, 1992). Typically completed in up to 15 minutes by a clinician or trained professional, it has been adapted into Spanish as the EB25. A validation study of 66 patients with mild dementia (26 AD, 12 VD, 4 MD, 23 FTD, 1 NSD) and 66 matched controls found high internal consistency ($\alpha = 0.87$), excellent test-retest (ICC = 0.89, 95% CI 0.76–0.91) and inter-rater reliability (ICC = 0.94), and strong correlations with other executive measures, though age differences between diagnostic subgroups limited interpretability (Serrani Azcurra, 2013).

Normative data for Mexican Americans were later established from a sample of 797 adults (mean age 60.4, 73.4% women, and mean education 9.9 years), with approximately half tested in Spanish (O'Bryant et al, 2018). Regression analyses revealed education as the strongest predictor of EXIT-25 performance (27% of variance), with gender explaining 4%. Norm tables were stratified by education (0–6, 3–9, 6–12, and 12+ years) and age (40–60 and 61+), though the authors cautioned against generalizing these norms to other Hispanic populations.

Strengths and Limitations: The EXIT-25 is a reliable and valid measure of executive dysfunction, showing high internal consistency ($\alpha = 0.87$), test–retest (ICC = 0.89), and inter-rater reliability (ICC = 0.94). It covers a broad range of executive domains, can be administered in under 15 minutes by trained professionals, and has normative data for Mexican Americans stratified by age and education, enhancing its clinical value. It effectively distinguishes between AD and FTD, with education emerging as the strongest performance predictor. However, its broader use is limited by small validation samples, a lack of norms beyond Mexican Americans, potential cultural/linguistic differences across Spanish-speaking groups, and the need for trained personnel for reliable administration.

Behavioral Inhibition Scale

The Behavioral Inhibition Scale (BIS) is a short, informant-rated questionnaire focusing on withdrawal-related traits such as self-criticism and social anxiety (Carver, 1994). Comprised of just seven items, it minimizes burden while retaining discriminatory potential between clinical groups. The BIS is available in Spanish through the National Alzheimer's Coordinating Center (NACC), though no normative data are published, and validation in Spanish-speaking populations has not been established.

Strengths and Limitations: The BIS's brevity and focus on clinically relevant withdrawal traits make it appealing for both clinical and research use, and the informant-based approach enables evaluation when patient self-report is unreliable. However, the absence of normative data, cutoff guidelines, and validation in Spanish-speaking populations severely constrains its interpretability. Psychometric evidence remains sparse overall, raising uncertainty about reliability and validity, and informant bias is a particular concern for subjective constructs like social anxiety. Substantial further validation is needed before widespread adoption.

Mild Behavioral Impairment Checklist

The Mild Behavioral Impairment Checklist (MBI-C) is a 34-item tool designed to detect emergent behavioral symptoms in individuals with mild cognitive impairment, organized into five domains: decreased motivation, affective dysregulation, impulse control, social inappropriateness, and abnormal thought/perception (Ismail et al, 2017). Items are rated for severity (1–3) and must reflect a meaningful change from baseline. A Spanish validation study in Santiago de Compostela examined 111 participants ≥50 years with MCI (mean age 70.04, SD = 8.33; mean education 7.89 years, and SD = 4.07), though sex/gender breakdown was not reported (Mallo et al, 2018). The optimal cutoff score of 6.5 yielded excellent sensitivity (100%) and good specificity (78.2%), with phone-based administration (10–15 minutes) proving feasible. The Spanish version was produced through back-translation for accuracy.

Strengths and Limitations: The MBI-C offers comprehensive domain coverage, clear severity scaling, and strong diagnostic accuracy for behavioral change in MCI, with additional advantages of phone administration and linguistic validation into Spanish. Its brevity (10–15 minutes) enhances feasibility across clinical and research settings. However, evidence rests on a single small study from Spain, with no validation in other Spanish-speaking populations and no reporting of gender distribution. The tool was originally designed for research, and comparative studies with other behavioral measures are lacking. Broader psychometric evaluation and cross-cultural validation are required before recommending widespread clinical use.

IMPACT OF BILINGUALISM, CULTURAL FACTORS, AND ACCULTURATION ON COGNITIVE ASSESSMENT

Cognitive assessment in older Hispanic/Latino migrants is shaped by the interplay of bilingualism, cultural factors, and acculturation. Bilingualism could affect cognitive testing through both advantages and challenges. While bilingualism has been associated with cognitive reserve and potential protective effects against age-related decline, it can also complicate neuropsychological assessment. Test performance may vary depending on the individual's dominant language, age of acquisition, proficiency in each language, and the language of test administration. Additionally, cultural factors such as familism, culturally specific beliefs, and positive and negative ethnic experiences could influence both symptom reporting and performance on standardized tasks. Acculturation, which refers to the process of adapting to a new cultural environment, has emerged as a key factor in understanding health outcomes among aging Hispanic/Latino populations in the U.S., including cognitive and brain aging. Research on the role of acculturation in cognitive aging has yielded inconsistent findings. Some studies associate lower acculturation (e.g., foreign nativity or Spanish language preference) with lower cognitive performance and dementia risk, while others suggest the opposite or no relationship at all. These discrepancies may stem from differences in how acculturation is measured (e.g., years in the U.S. or age at migration) and how it interacts with moderating factors like sex, cognitive status, and socioeconomic background.

Given these challenges, cognitive assessments must include validated measures of acculturation, familism, ethnic experiences, and bilingualism to contextualize performance, distinguish between normative cultural-linguistic variation and true impairment, and ensure diagnostic accuracy. Incorporating these measures allows for more culturally responsive evaluation practices and reduces the risk of misclassification in older Latino migrant populations.

ASSESSMENT OF BILINGUALISM

Linguistic History Questionnaire (CLS) (UDSv3)

The Language History Questionnaire (LHQ) is a self-report measure of linguistic background and proficiency in bilinguals and multilinguals. Developed from a review of 41 published studies, it consolidates the most commonly assessed variables, including age of language acquisition, length of residence in the U.S., and proficiency in reading, writing, speaking, and comprehension (Li, Sepanski, and Zhao, 2006). The updated LHQ3 retains 22 online questions but adds an improved interface and scoring system, covering three domains:

- Proficiency, based on weighted self-ratings across listening, speaking, reading, and writing
- Immersion, calculated from age, age of acquisition, and years of use
- Dominance, scored from hours of daily use and relative self-rated proficiency (Li, 2020)

Evidence for construct validity comes from the use of previously validated questions and from empirical testing. In a study of 40 English-Spanish bilingual undergraduates at the University of Richmond (17 males, 23 females, ages 18–22; M age of Spanish acquisition = 11.7, SD = 3.9), the LHQ demonstrated predictive and discriminative validity, as well as split-half reliability, when compared against sentence comprehension tasks and verbal SAT scores (Sepanski, 2007).

Strengths and Limitations: The LHQ is comprehensive, customizable, low-cost, and easily administered online, making it efficient for large-scale or targeted studies of bilingualism, heritage language use, and second-language acquisition. However, as a self-report instrument, it is subject to recall and self-assessment bias, with potential cultural and educational influences on responses. While it offers valuable multidimensional data, it is best complemented by objective proficiency tests or qualitative methods for a fuller picture of an individual's language profile.

NP-NUMBRS Fluency Ratio (FAS/PMR)

The Neuropsychological Norms for the U.S.-Mexico Border Region in Spanish (NP-NUMBRS) project established normative data for two verbal fluency tasks in native Spanish speakers residing in or near the U.S.-Mexico border, specifically San Diego, California, and Tucson, Arizona (Marquine, Morlett Paredes et al, 2021). The study included 254 adults ages 19–60 years (M = 37.32, SD = 10.24), all of whom completed a comprehensive neuropsychological battery. Verbal fluency was assessed through two tasks. In the letter fluency task, participants were asked to generate words beginning with the letters P, M, and R, with 60 seconds allotted for each letter; proper names, plurals, and repetitions were excluded, and performance was scored based on the number of correct words produced. In the semantic fluency task, participants named as many animals as possible within 60 seconds, again with intrusions and repetitions excluded.

The study examined whether norms developed for other cultural and linguistic groups could be applied to Spanish speakers and compared impairment classification rates from existing published norms with those derived from the new NP-NUMBRS data. The findings showed that applying non-Spanish norms produced significant demographic effects on test performance, often misclassifying Spanish-speaking individuals as impaired due to cultural and linguistic differences rather than true cognitive deficits. In contrast, the newly established, demographically adjusted norms offered a more accurate framework, with performance on both fluency tasks positively associated with education and age.

Strengths and Limitations: The FAS/PMR ratio can reveal subtle cognitive-linguistic differences not evident in raw fluency scores, but it is highly influenced by demographic factors such as age, education, and language background. Therefore, its interpretation should always be grounded in the individual's broader language history, cognitive profile, and sociodemographic context.

Language Experience and Proficiency Questionnaire

The Language Experience and Proficiency Questionnaire (LEAP-Q) is a validated self-report tool for assessing language proficiency and experience in bilinguals and multilinguals (Marian, Blumenfeld, and Kaushanskaya, 2007). It consists of two parts with a total of 16 items (9 and 7, respectively) and integrates measures of language competence, acquisition, and exposure. Language competence is captured through proficiency ratings in speaking, listening, reading, and writing, along with self-reported dominance and language preference. Acquisition history is assessed through the ages of first learning, fluency, reading, and reading fluency, as well as the contexts in which each language was acquired. Language exposure and use are evaluated across environments such as home, school, work, and country of residence, as well as current use with family, friends, and media.

The validity of the LEAP-Q was established over two studies. Study 1 established internal validity with 52 bilinguals (M = 27.29, SD = 5.92; 29 women, 23 men) from Northwestern University and the Chicago area, whose responses informed refinement of the instrument. Study 2 further confirmed its validity with a more homogeneous sample of 50 English-Spanish bilinguals (M = 26.7, SD = 10.4; 31 women, 19 men), including 18 native Spanish and 32 native English speakers. Participants completed standardized behavioral language tests after completing the LEAP-Q, supporting its reliability and validity as a measure of bilingual language status (Marian, Blumenfeld, and Kaushanskaya, 2007).

> **Strengths and Limitations:** The LEAP-Q provides detailed, multidimensional data on language background, is cost-free, digital, and easy to administer online, and allows both qualitative and quantitative analyses. However, as a self-report tool, it is vulnerable to biases in self-assessment and to cultural or educational differences in how questions are interpreted, which may affect data reliability.

ASSESSMENT OF ACCULTURATION

Short Acculturation Scale for Hispanics

The Short Acculturation Scale for Hispanics (SASH) (Marín et al, 1987) is a 12-item self-administered measure designed to assess acculturation levels among Hispanics in the United States. The scale is divided into three subscales and demonstrates high internal reliability (Cronbach's $\alpha = .92$):

- Language use (five items)
- Media use (three items)
- Ethnic social relations (four items)

Development of the SASH was based on a sample of 591 participants recruited primarily in San Francisco, with additional participants from Florida and Wisconsin. The sample included 228 non-Hispanic Whites (M = 38.8 years; 57% female) and 363 Hispanics (M = 31.2 years; 62% female), of whom 70% were foreign-born. Hispanic subgroups consisted of Mexican Americans (n = 160), Cuban Americans (n = 21), Puerto Ricans (n = 7), and other Hispanics (n = 175). On average, immigrant participants had resided in the U.S. for 14.7 years (range = 15–75, SD = 11.56).

Participants completed a 16-page questionnaire in English or Spanish, which included demographic items, cultural values, and an initial 17-item version of the SASH. Items were adapted from existing acculturation measures and reworded for clarity to capture language proficiency and preference, media consumption, and preferred ethnicity of social contacts. The final 12 items were selected for their strong psychometric properties.

Validity of the SASH was supported through correlations with generational status, length of residence, acculturative index, and age of arrival, as well as by comparing participants' SASH scores with their self-rated acculturation. Across all criteria, results indicated significantly positive associations, establishing the scale as a reliable and valid measure of behavioral acculturation. While few longitudinal studies exist assessing change in SASH scores over time, those that do suggest that social and language-based acculturation are relatively stable across U.S.-based populations (Lamar et al, 2023) including the Boston Puerto Rican Health study (Vercammen et al, 2019).

Strengths and Limitations: The SASH is a brief, reliable, and practical tool that captures key aspects of acculturation, including language, media, and social relations, showing strong internal consistency and validity. Its bilingual format increases accessibility across Hispanic populations. However, its development from a geographically limited and unevenly represented sample reduces generalizability, and its focus on behavior may neglect broader cultural dimensions such as identity and values.

The Acculturation Scale for Mexican Americans

The Acculturation Rating Scale for Mexican Americans-II (ARSMA-II) (Cuéllar, 1995) is a revision of the original unidimensional measure, reconceptualized as a bidimensional scale to capture the four modes of acculturation: integration, separation, assimilation, and marginalization. The 30-item scale includes two primary subscales, the Anglo Orientation Subscale (AOS) and the Mexican Orientation Subscale (MOS), with an optional 18-item Marginality Scale comprising Anglo, Mexican, and Mexican American marginality subscales. The ARSMA-II assesses four cultural domains: language use and preference, ethnic identity and classification, cultural heritage and behaviors, and ethnic interaction.

The measure was validated with 379 participants in Texas (23% Mexican, 58% Mexican American, 11% White non-Hispanic; 48% female) and demonstrated strong internal reliability for both the AOS (.86) and MOS (.88). Construct validity was supported through high correlations with the original ARSMA ($r = .89$), while the Marginality Scale also showed strong reliability ($\alpha = .87$).

Strengths and Limitations: The ARSMA-II is a reliable, valid tool that assesses Mexican and Anglo cultural orientations separately, offering a nuanced view of acculturation across language, identity, practices, and social interactions. However, its development with Mexican-origin samples in Texas limits generalizability, and the optional Marginality Scale, though reliable, may be less practical due to added length.

Scale of Ethnic Experience

The Scale of Ethnic Experience (SEE) (Malcarne et al, 2006) is a 32-item self-report instrument designed to assess four domains of ethnicity-related cognition across groups: Ethnic Identity, Perceived Discrimination, Mainstream Comfort, and Social Affiliation. The scale was developed and refined across five studies, beginning with qualitative item generation and focus groups, which narrowed an initial pool of 100 items to a 73-item pilot version. Factor analysis with a diverse student sample ($N = 638$) identified four reliable factors, resulting in the final 32-item scale. Subsequent studies demonstrated strong internal consistency, six-week test-retest reliability (r = .77–86), concurrent validity with existing measures of ethnic identity and acculturation, and cross-validated factor structure in a larger, ethnically diverse sample (N = 940).

Strengths and Limitations: The SEE is a reliable, validated measure that captures both positive (identity, affiliation) and negative (discrimination) aspects of ethnic experience across diverse groups, making it more comprehensive than many unidimensional tools. However, its reliance on college student samples limits generalizability, and it may overlook cultural nuances within specific groups.

Psychological Acculturation Scale

The Psychological Acculturation Scale (PAS) (Tropp et al, 1999) is a 10-item bilingual measure designed to assess four psychological dimensions of acculturation: cultural loyalty, solidarity, identification, and comprehension. Items address beliefs, confidence, and cultural knowledge using a nine-point Likert scale. Validation was conducted across three studies. In Study 1, 36 bilingual Latinos (28% male, 72% female; ages 14–58; 13 U.S.-born, 23 foreign-born) completed both English and Spanish versions, yielding strong cross-language consistency (total score r = .94; item-level r = .83–.85). In Study 2, 107 Puerto Ricans (ages 12–58; 39 male, 64 female, 4 missing) completed the PAS in their preferred language, showing high internal consistency (English α = .83; Spanish α = .90) and strong associations with cultural behavior and preference items. Study 3 extended validation to different age groups, including 247 Puerto Rican adolescents (ages 3–14; 118 male, 129 female) and 228 mothers (ages 27–57; M = 39), using interview administration alongside migration and demographic data. Results indicated that psychological acculturation was more strongly related to cultural behaviors and preferences than length of residence in the U.S., supporting the PAS as a reliable and valid measure across languages and age groups.

Strengths and Limitations: The PAS is a reliable, bilingual tool that captures psychological aspects of acculturation including loyalty, identification, solidarity, and comprehension, beyond simple demographic indicators. Its strengths include strong cross-language reliability and validation across age groups, but its testing has been limited mainly to Hispanic/Latino populations, and it does not account for behavioral or structural aspects of acculturation.

Abbreviated Multidimensional Acculturation Scale Hispanic-American Version

The Abbreviated Multidimensional Acculturation Scale (AMAS-ZABB) (Zea et al, 2003) is a bilinear, multidimensional measure designed for adaptability across cultures. It consists of 42 items, 21 each for the culture of origin and host culture, covering three domains: cultural identity (6 items), language competence (9 items), and cultural competence (6 items). Responses use 4-point Likert scales, ranging from strongly disagree to strongly agree for identity, and from not at all to extremely well/like a native for language and cultural competence. An initial 80-item version was piloted with Hispanic/Latino and immigrant participants, and refined to the current 42-item form.

Validation was conducted across two studies. Study 1, with 156 Latino college students (M = 23.49, SD = 7.41; ~60% female), demonstrated strong internal consistency (α = .90–.97). Concurrent validity was supported by significant differences between U.S.-born and foreign-born participants, and by correlations between length of residence and acculturation scores: English language use and U.S. cultural competence increased with residence, whereas Spanish language use, Hispanic/Latino identity, and cultural competence decreased. Study 2, using 90 Central American immigrants (M = 38.92, SD = 14.23; 52% female), confirmed high reliability (α = .83–97) and cross-validation with the Bicultural Involvement Questionnaire-Short Version BIQ-B and the Multi-Ethnic Identity Measure (MEIM) (Phinney, 1992). Results indicated independence between English and Spanish language competence, further supporting the bilinear structure.

Strengths and Limitations: The AMAS-ZABB is a reliable, multidimensional tool that captures both heritage and host cultures across identity, language, and cultural competence, offering a comprehensive view of biculturalism. Its strengths include strong psychometric support and adaptability, but as a self-report measure, it is prone to bias and does not account for changes in acculturation over time or context-specific cultural nuances.

Sabogal Familism Scale

The Sabogal Familism Scale (Sabogal, 1987) is a 14-item questionnaire developed to assess three dimensions of familism: familial obligations, family support, and family as referents. It was validated with 452 Hispanics and 227 White non-Hispanics in San Francisco and Miami, using both English and Spanish versions. Items assessed attitudinal familism, behavioral acculturation, and demographics, with responses recorded on a 5-point Likert scale (1 = very much in disagreement to 5 = very much in agreement). Results indicated that familism dimensions were inversely related to the level of acculturation, a relationship that held even when controlling for sociodemographic factors, applying different acculturation criteria, and examining across Hispanic/Latino subgroups. These findings supported the role of familism as a central cultural value within Hispanic/Latino populations.

Strengths and Limitations: The Sabogal Familism Scale is a culturally grounded, bilingual measure that reliably captures obligations, support, and family as referents, and has been widely validated across Hispanic/Latino groups. However, as a self-report tool, it is prone to bias and may not fully capture generational or contextual shifts in family dynamics; in fact, reports suggest that changes in familism previously documented in younger Latinos Cruz et al. (2021) are also noted in older Latinos (Lamar et al, 2023).

Hispanic Stress Inventory (Foreign-Born, United States-Born Forms)

The Hispanic Stress Inventory (HSI) and its immigrant version (HSI-I) (Cervantes, 1991) were developed to provide a culturally appropriate measure of psychosocial stress among Hispanics. The final scales include 73 items across five domains:

- Acculturation stress (40 items)
- Family stress (40 items)
- Perceived discrimination (19 items)
- Occupational/economic stress (18 items)
- Marital stress (16 items)

Responses are rated on a 5-point Likert scale. Development involved four stages: item generation, content validation, construct validation, and reliability testing. Item development began with interviews of 105 adult Hispanics, yielding 176 potential items, which were later refined to 133 after expert review for cultural relevance. Construct validity was tested with 493 Hispanics (305 immigrants, 188 U.S.-born), who completed the inventory in English or Spanish. Analyses supported distinct immigrant and U.S.-born versions of the scale, reflecting different stress profiles. Internal consistency was high, with subscale alphas ranging from .77–.91, and test-retest reliability with 35 adults showed coefficients between r = .61–.86, confirming stability over time.

Further validation was provided by Cavazos-Rehg (2006), who developed an abbreviated 25-item HSI-I tested on 143 Latino immigrants (M = 37 years, SD = 10.66; 80 females, 63 males) in St. Louis. This version retained the five-factor structure, including occupational/economic stress, parental stress, marital stress, immigration stress, and family/culture stress, and demonstrated support for validity, with item-factor loadings and correlations ranging from r = .175–.302.

Strengths and Limitations: The HSI and HSI-I offer important strengths, including culturally tailored content that distinguishes stressors faced by immigrant and U.S.-born Hispanics, such as immigration challenges, language barriers, discrimination, and intergenerational conflict. Both the full and abbreviated versions have demonstrated strong reliability and validity, with high internal consistency and stable test-retest results, making them useful in both clinical and research settings. However, as self-report instruments, they are subject to social desirability and underreporting biases, and they may not fully capture dynamic or context-specific stressors that evolve over time.

CLINICAL AND RESEARCH APPLICATIONS

This book offers a comprehensive review of Spanish-language neuropsychological assessments for older Latino/Hispanic populations, addressing a critical need for culturally and linguistically appropriate cognitive testing. It assists clinicians in selecting instruments that are psychometrically sound and normed for Spanish-speaking older adults, thereby reducing diagnostic errors associated with language, cultural, and educational differences. The text provides detailed guidance on test selection, including information on sample characteristics and normative data, and offers recommendations for choosing appropriate measures across cognitive domains such as memory, language, and attention. Moreover, the book underscores the importance of considering factors such as bilingualism, acculturation, and literacy in the neuropsychological evaluation process to promote valid and equitable assessment outcomes. It also includes tools for evaluating functional abilities and assessing the influence of psychiatric or psychological symptoms on cognitive performance.

Clinicians should nonetheless recognize that selecting an appropriate neuropsychological measure requires careful consideration of multiple factors to ensure that the assessment is clinically meaningful, psychometrically robust, and culturally appropriate for the individual being evaluated. The following factors should be considered:

1. **Clarify the referral question.**
   Determine the purpose of the assessment. Is it for differential diagnosis (e.g., dementia versus depression), to document cognitive decline, assess functional impact, or monitor treatment progress? The referral question guides which cognitive domains to prioritize and the depth of the evaluation.

2. **Consider the patient's background.**
   Understand the individual's linguistic, cultural, and educational context. Is the person monolingual, bilingual, or multilingual? Were they raised and educated outside the U.S.? What was the quality of their formal education? Are there test norms available for their age, education level, and cultural background? Matching the patient to appropriate normative data is essential for valid interpretation.

3. **Match tests to cognitive domains.**
   The book organizes tests by domain (e.g., memory, language, executive function), allowing clinicians to select instruments based on the specific areas of concern.
4. **Evaluate psychometric properties.**
   Choose tests that are both reliable and valid for the target population. Strong psychometric properties, including sensitivity and specificity, enhance the accuracy of clinical decisions.
5. **Consider practical factors.**
   Consider administration time, test availability (commercial versus open access), and the patient's cognitive capacity to tolerate the test length. Choose tools that are feasible for the patient and the clinical setting.
6. **Include functional and validity measures.**
   Assess real-world functioning using validated functional scales (e.g., ADLs, IADLs), and if needed, ensure test results are credible by including performance and symptom validity measures.

Beyond clinical practice, the book serves as a critical resource for neuropsychological researchers. It aids in the following:

- Selecting culturally valid tools for studies involving older Spanish-speaking populations enhances the accuracy and interpretability of research findings.
- Supporting normative data development, highlighting current efforts in the U.S., Latin America, and Spain to produce population-specific norms.
- Enabling cross-national and cross-linguistic comparisons by detailing psychometric properties across diverse Spanish-speaking groups.
- Identifying limitations in existing tools, encouraging further research to address gaps and improving test development and validation.

CONCLUSIONS AND FUTURE DIRECTIONS

Given the disproportionate burden of dementia among Latino/Hispanic older adults in the U.S., ensuring the cultural and linguistic appropriateness of cognitive assessments is both urgent and essential. Accurate diagnosis of conditions like MCI and dementia depends heavily on neuropsychological test performance, underscoring the importance of validated tools with robust psychometric properties. Our review, led by the CADLAS Cognition and Assessment group, highlights both the strengths and limitations of currently available Spanish-language tests for individuals aged >55 years. While some tests have demonstrated reliability and utility across diverse Spanish-speaking populations, inconsistencies in sampling, norming procedures, and cultural considerations limit their generalizability and clinical utility.

Future research must prioritize the development and validation of cognitive measures in larger, more diverse Spanish-speaking samples, with attention to rural versus urban populations, varying educational and socioeconomic backgrounds. Develop norms that account for bilingualism, biculturalism, and sociocultural diversity beyond the country of origin or language. Cross-national comparisons of test performance and culturally sensitive adaptations are also needed to better understand how linguistic and cultural context influence cognitive assessment. Increase collaboration between U.S. and Latin American researchers to harmonize data collection and interpretation. Encourage longitudinal studies of cognitive aging and dementia progression in Latino/Hispanic populations using culturally valid instruments. Validate technology-based cognitive assessments in Spanish-speaking populations with varying levels of digital literacy. Explore the potential of digital tools and telehealth in increasing access to culturally appropriate testing in underserved Latino communities. Finally, combine cognitive testing with biomarkers (e.g., blood-based markers, neuroimaging) to enhance diagnostic precision and understand disease mechanisms in diverse populations. As the Latino/Hispanic older adult population continues to grow, investment in inclusive and equitable diagnostic tools will be critical for improving early detection and care outcomes across diverse communities.

REFERENCES

Abbott, RA, Skirrow, C, Jokisch, M, et al. Normative data from linear and nonlinear quantile regression in CANTAB: Cognition in mid-to-late life in an epidemiological sample. *Alzheimer's & Dementia (Amsterdam, Netherlands)*. 2019; 11: 36–44.

Acevedo, AKR, Krueger, E, Navarro, F, et al. The Spanish translation and adaptation of the Uniform Data Set of the National Institute on Aging Alzheimer's Disease Centers. *Alzheimer's Disease & Associated Disorders*. 2009; 23: 102–9.

Aguilar-Navarro, SG, Mimenza-Alvarado, AJ, Palacios-Garcia, AA, et al. Validity and reliability of the Spanish version of the Montreal Cognitive Assessment (MoCA) for the detection of cognitive impairment in Mexico. *Revista Colombiana de Psiquiatría* (English edition). 2018; 47: 237–43.

Aguilar-Navarro, SG, Sanchez, BLP,Gutierrez, LAG, et al. Cross-cultural adaptation of the everyday cognition scale (M-ECog) in older Mexican adults with cognitive impairment. *Dementia & Neuropsychologia*. 2023; 17: e20230011.

Aguirre-Acevedo, DC, Gómez, RD, Moreno, S, et al. Validez y fiabilidad de la batería neuropsicológica CERAD-Col. *Revista de Neurología*. 2007; 45: 655–60.

Ahmed, I, Ishtiaq, S. Reliability and validity: Importance in medical research. *JPMA. The Journal of the Pakistan Medical Association*. 2021; 71: 2401–06.

Alegret, MN, Munoz, N, Roberto, DM, et al. A computerized version of the Short Form of the Face-Name Associative Memory Exam (FACEmemory®) for the early detection of Alzheimer's disease. *Alzheimer's Research & Therapy*. 2020; 12:25.

Alegret, MS, Valero, G, Ortega, A, et al. Validation of the Spanish Version of the Face Name Associative Memory Exam (S-FNAME) in Cognitively Normal Older Individuals. *Archives of Clinical Neuropsychology*. 2015; 30: 712–20.

Alviarez-Schulze, V, Cattaneo, G, Pachon-Garcia, C, et al. Validation and normative data of the Spanish version of the Face Name Associative Memory Exam (S-FNAME). *Journal of the International Neuropsychological Society*. 2022; 28: 74–84.

Andreu, Y, Galdon, MJ, Dura, E, et al. Psychometric properties of the Brief Symptoms Inventory-18 (BSI-18) in a Spanish sample of outpatients with psychiatric disorders. *Psicothema*. 2008; 20: 844–50.

Arango-Lasprilla, JC. Commonly used neuropsychological tests for Spanish speakers: Normative data from Latin America. *NeuroRehabilitation*. 2015; 37: 489–91.

Arango-Lasprilla, JC, Ayearst, LE, Rivera, D, et al. Test of memory Malingering. 2nd ed: Normative data from cognitively intact adults living in Spain. *Applied Neuropsychology Adult*. 2024; 1–7.

Arango-Lasprilla, JC, Rivera, D, Aguayo, A, et al. Trail Making Test: Normative data for the Latin American Spanish speaking adult population. *NeuroRehabilitation*. 2015; 37: 639–61.

Arango-Lasprilla, JC, Rivera, D, Garza, MT, et al. Hopkins Verbal Learning Test – Revised: Normative data for the Latin American Spanish speaking adult population. *NeuroRehabilitation*. 2015; 37: 699–718.

Arango-Lasprilla, JC, Rivera, D, Longoni, M, et al. Modified Wisconsin card sorting test (M-WCST): Normative data for the Latin American Spanish speaking adult population. *NeuroRehabilitation*. 2015; 37: 563–90.

Arango-Lasprilla, JC, Rivera, D, Rodríguez, G, et al. Symbol digit modalities test: Normative data for the Latin American Spanish speaking adult population. *NeuroRehabilitation*. 2015; 37: 625–38.

Arango-Lasprilla, JC, Rivera, D, Rodriguez, MJ. WHO-UCLA auditory verbal learning test: Normative data for Spanish-speaking adults in the United States. *NeuroRehabilitation*. 2024; 55: 183–93.

Ardila, A, Rosselli, M, Puente, AE. *Critical Issues in Neuropsychology: Neuropsychological Evaluation of the Spanish Speaker.* Plenum Press, New York, NY, U.S.: 1994.

Arevalo-Rodriguez, I, Smailagic, N, Figuls, I, et al. Mini-Mental State Examination (MMSE) for the detection of Alzheimer's disease and other dementias in people with mild cognitive impairment (MCI). *The Cochrane Database of Systematic Reviews*. 2015: CD010783.

Artiola i Fortuny, L, Heaton, RK, Hermosillo, D. Neuropsychological comparisons of Spanish-speaking participants from the U.S.-Mexico border region versus Spain. *Journal of the International Neuropsychological Society*. 1998; 4: 363–79.

Artiola i Fortuny, L, Heaton, RK. Standard versus computerized administration of the Wisconsin Card Sorting Test. *Clinical Neuropsychologist*. 1996; 10: 419–24.

Artiola i Fortuny, L, Romo, DH, Heaton, RK, et al. *Manual de Normas y Procedimientos para la Batería Neuropsicológica en Español.* [Manual of Norms and Procedures for the Spanish Neuropsychological Battery.] Pardee Press, Tuscon, AZ, U.S.: 1999.

Baker, FM and Espino, DV. A Spanish version of the geriatric depression scale in Mexican-American elders. *International Journal of Geriatric Psychiatry*. 1997; 12: 21–5.

Beaumont, JL, Havlik, R, Cook, KF, et al. Norming plans for the NIH Toolbox. *Neurology*.2013; 80: S87–92.

Beck, AT, Steer, RA, and Brown, GK. Beck Depression Inventory-II manual. The Psychological Corporation, San Antonio, TX, U.S.: 1996

Beck, AT, Steer, RA, Brown, GK. Beck Anxiety Inventory Manual: The Psychological Corporation, Harcourt Brace & Co., San Antonio, TX, U.S.: 1993.

Benedict, RHB, Groninger, L. Preliminary standardization of a new visuospatial memory test with six alternate forms. *The Clinical Neuropsychologist*. 1995; 9: 11–16.

Benedict, RHB, Schretlen, D, Groninger, L, et al. Revision of the Brief Visuospatial Memory Test: Studies of normal performance, reliability, and validity. *Psychological Assessment*. 1996; 8: 145–52.

Benedict, RHB, Schretlen, D, Groninger, L, et al. Hopkins Verbal Learning Test–Revised: Normative data and analysis of inter-form and test-retest reliability. *The Clinical Neuropsychologist*, 1998; 12: 43–55.

Benedict, RHB, Smerbeck, A, Parikh, R, et al. Reliability and equivalence of alternate forms for the Symbol Digit Modalities Test: Implications for multiple sclerosis clinical trials. *Multiple Sclerosis Journal*, 2012; 18: 1320–25.

Benson, G, de Felipe, J, Xiaodong, et al. Performance of Spanish-speaking community-dwelling elders in the United States on the Uniform Data Set. *Alzheimer's & Dementia*. 2014; 10: S338–43.

Benton, AL. Problems of test construction in the field of aphasia. *Cortex: A Journal Devoted to the Study of the Nervous System and Behavior*. 1967; 3: 32–58.

Benton, AL, Sivan, AB, Hamsher, K. *Contributions to Neuropsychological Assessment: A Clinical Manual.* (2nd ed.). Oxford University Press, New York, NY, U.S.: 1994.

Benton, AL, Hamsher, K. *Multilingual Aphasia Examination Manual.* University of Iowa, Iowa City, IA: 1976.

Benton, AL, Hamsher, K, Sivan, AB. *Multilingual aphasia examination* (3rd ed.). AJA Associates, Iowa City, IA: 1983.

Benton, AL, Varney, NR, Hamsher, K. Judgment of line orientation [database record]. *APA PsycTests, Washington DC,* U.S.: 1975.

Boada, M, Cejudo JC, Tarraga, L, et al. Neuropsychiatric inventory questionnaire (NPI-Q): Spanish validation of an abridged form of the Neuropsychiatric Inventory (NPI)]. *Neurología*. 2002; 17: 317–23.

Bonete-López, B, Oltra-Cucarella, J, Marín, M, et al. Validation and Norms for a Recognition Task for the Spanish Version of the Free and Cued Selective Reminding Test. *Archives of Clinical Neuropsychology*. 2020; 36: 954–64.

Boone, KB, Salazar, X, Lu, P, et al. The Rey 15-item recognition trial: A technique to enhance sensitivity of the Rey 15-item memorization test. *Journal of Clinical and Experimental Neuropsychology*. 24: 561–73.

Bors, DA, and Stokes, TL. Raven's Advanced Progressive Matrices: Norms for first-year university students and the development of a short form. *Educational and Psychological Measurement*. 1998; 58: 382–98.

Borson, S, Scanlan J, Brush, M, et al. The mini-cog: A cognitive "vital signs" measure for dementia screening in multi-lingual elderly. *International Journal of Geriatric Psychiatry*. 2000; 15: 1021–7.

Bowler, RM, Thaler, DA,and Rauch, SS. Digit Symbol and Symbol Digit Modalities Tests: A comparison of two coding tasks. *Neuropsychology*. 1992; 6: 327–35.

Breton, J, Stickel, AM, Tarraf, W, et al. Normative data for the Brief Spanish-English Verbal Learning Test for representative and diverse Hispanics/Latinos: Results from the Hispanic Community Health Study/Study of Latinos (HCHS/SOL). *Alzheimer's & Dementia (Amsterdam, Netherlands)*. 2021; 13: e12260.

Brugulat-Serrat, A, Cañas-Martínez, A, Canals-Gispert, L, et al. Enhancing the sensitivity of memory tests: Reference data for the Free and Cued Selective Reminding Test and the Logical Memory Task from cognitively healthy subjects with normal Alzheimer's disease cerebrospinal fluid biomarker levels. *Journal of Alzheimer's Disease*. 2021; 84: 119–28.

Bruno, D, Slachevsky, A, Fiorentino, N, et al. Argentinian/Chilean validation of the Spanish-language version of Addenbrooke's Cognitive Examination III for diagnosing dementia. *Neurología (English Edition)*. 2020; 35: 82–88.

Buela-Casal, G, and Guillén-Riquelme, A. Short form of the Spanish adaptation of the State-Trait Anxiety Inventory. *International Journal of Clinical and Health Psychology*. 2017; 17(3): 261-68.

Bugallo-Carrera, C, Dosil-Diaz, C, Pereiro, AX, et al. Assessment of validity and comparison of two Spanish versions of the Geriatric Depression Scale. *Frontiers in Psychology*. 2023; 14: 1101886.

Burin, DI, Jorge, RE, Arizaga, RA, et al. Estimation of premorbid intelligence: The word accentuation test – Buenos Aires version. *Journal of Clinical and Experimental Neuropsychology*. 2000; 22: 677–85.

Burke, SL, Naseh, M, Rodriguez, MJ, et al. Dementia-related neuropsychological testing considerations in non-Hispanic white and Latino/Hispanic populations. *Psychology & Neuroscience*. 2019; 12: 144–68.

Buschke, H. Cued recall in amnesia. *Journal of Clinical Neuropsychology*. 1984; 6: 433–40.

Buschke, H, Kuslansky, G, Katz, M, et al. Screening for dementia with the memory impairment screen. *Neurology*. 1999; 52: 231–8.

Callahan, CM, Unverzagt, FW, Hui, SL, et al. Six-item screener to identify cognitive impairment among potential subjects for clinical research. *Medical Care*. 2002; 40: 771–81.

Calvo, L, Casals-Coll, M, Sanchez-Benavides, G, et al. Spanish normative studies in young adults (NEURONORMA young adults project): Norms for the Visual Object and Space Perception Battery and Judgment of Line Orientation tests. *Neurología*. 2013; 28: 153–9.

Campo, P, Morales, M. Normative data and reliability for a Spanish version of the verbal Selective Reminding Test. *Archives of Clinical Neuropsychology*. 2004; 19: 421–35.

Campo, P, Morales, M and Juan-Malpartida, M. Development of two Spanish versions of the verbal Selective Reminding Test. *Journal of Clinical and Experimental Neuropsychology*. 2000; 22: 279–85.

Campos-Magdaleno, M, Nieto-Vieites, A, Frades-Payo, B, et al. Normative data for the Spanish versions of the CVLT, WMS-Logical Memory, and RBMT from a sample of middle-aged and old participants. *Psychological Assessment*. 2024; 36: 114.

Carnero-Pardo, C, Cruz-Orduna, I, Espejo-Martinez, B, et al. Utility of the Mini-Cog for detection of cognitive impairment in primary care: Data from two Spanish studies. *International Journal of Alzheimer's Disease*. 2013: 285462.

Carnero-Pardo, C, Rego-Garcia, I, Mene Llorente, M, et al. Diagnostic performance of brief cognitive tests in cognitive impairment screening. *Neurología (English Edition)*. 2022; 37: 441–49.

Carpenter, PA, Just, MA, Shell, P. What one intelligence test measures: A theoretical account of the processing in the Raven Progressive Matrices Test. *Psychological Review*. 1990; 97: 404.

Carrete, P, Augustovski, F, Gimpel, N, et al. Validation of a telephone-administered Geriatric Depression Scale in a Hispanic elderly population. *Journal of General Internal Medicine*. 2001; 16: 446–50.

Carrión, CI, Rivera, D, Forte, A, et al. Attention and processing speed tests: Normative data for Spanish-speaking adults in the United States. *NeuroRehabilitation*. 2024; 55: 169–82.

Carrion-Baralt, JR, Melendez-Cabrero, J, Schnaider Beeri, M, et al. The neuropsychological performance of nondemented Puerto Rican nonagenarians. *Dementia and Geriatric Cognitive Disorders*. 2009; 27: 353–60.

Carver, CS, White, TL. Behavioral inhibition, behavioral activation, and affective responses to impending reward and punishment: The BIS/BAS Scales. *Journal of Personality and Social Psychology*. 1994; 67: 319–33.

Casaletto, KB, Umlauf, A, Beaumont, J, et al. Demographically corrected normative standards for the English version of the NIH Toolbox Cognition Battery. *Journal of the International Neuropsychological Society*. 2015; 21: 378–91.

Casaletto, KB, Umlauf, A, Marquine, M, et al. Demographically Corrected Normative Standards for the Spanish Language Version of the NIH Toolbox Cognition Battery. *Journal of the International Neuropsychological Society*. 2016; 22: 364–74.

Cavazos-Rehg, PA, Zayas, LH, Walker, MS, et al. Evaluating an abbreviated version of the Hispanic Stress Inventory for Immigrants. *Hispanic Journal of Behavioral Sciences*. 2006; 28: 498–515.

Cervantes, RC, Padilla, AM, Salgado de Snyder, N. The Hispanic Stress Inventory: A culturally relevant approach to psychosocial assessment. *Psychological Assessment: A Journal of Consulting and Clinical Psychology*. 1991; 3: 438–47.

Chávez-Oliveros, M, Rodríguez-Agudelo, Y, Acosta-Castillo, I, et al. Semantic verbal fluency in elderly Mexican adults: Reference values. *Neurología (English Edition)*. 2015; 30: 189–94.

Cherner, M, Suarez, P, Lazzaretto, D, et al. Demographically corrected norms for the Brief Visuospatial Memory Test-revised and Hopkins Verbal Learning Test-revised in monolingual Spanish speakers from the U.S.–Mexico border region. *Archives of Clinical Neuropsychology*. 2007; 22: 343–53.

Cherner, M, Marquine, MJ, Umlauf, A, et al. Neuropsychological Norms for the U.S.-Mexico Border Region in Spanish (NP-NUMBRS) Project: Methodology and sample characteristics. *The Clinical Neuropsychologist*. 2021; 35: 253–68.

Contador, I, Bermejo-Pareja, F, Fernandez-Calvo, B, et al. The 37-item Version of the Mini-Mental State Examination: Normative data in a population-based cohort of older Spanish adults (NEDICES). *Archives of Clinical Neuropsychology*. 2016; 31: 263–72.

Corsi, PM. *Human Memory and the medial temporal region of the brain*. McGill University, Montreal, Canada: 1972.

Corwin, J, Bylsma, FW. Psychological examination of traumatic encephalopathy. *Clinical Neuropsychologist*. 1993; 7: 3–21.

Craft, S, Newcomer, J, Kanne, S, et al. Memory improvement following induced hyperinsulinemia in Alzheimer's disease. *Neurobiology of Aging*. 1996; 17: 123–30.

Crocco, EA, Loewenstein, DA, Curiel, RE, et al. A novel cognitive assessment paradigm to detect Pre-mild cognitive impairment (PreMCI) and the relationship to biological markers of Alzheimer's disease. *Journal of Psychiatric Research*. 2018; 96: 33–38.

Crocco, E, Curiel, RE, Acevedo, A, et al. An evaluation of deficits in semantic cueing and proactive and retroactive interference as early features of Alzheimer's disease. *The American Journal of Geriatric Psychiatry*. 2014; 22: 889–97.

Cruz, RA, Navarro, C, Carrera, K, et al. Mexican-origin youths' trajectories of internalizing symptoms from childhood into adolescence and associations with acculturation processes. *Journal of Clinical Child & Adolescent Psychology*. 2021; 50: 118–30.

Cuéllar, I, Arnold, B, Maldonado, R. Acculturation Rating Scale for Mexican Americans-II: A revision of the original ARSMA Scale. *Hispanic Journal of Behavioral Sciences*. 1995; 17: 275–304.

Cummings, JL, Mega, M, Gray, K, et al. The Neuropsychiatric Inventory: Comprehensive assessment of psychopathology in dementia. *Neurology*. 1994; 44: 2308–14.

Curiel Cid, RE, Crocco, EA, Duara, R, et al. A novel method of evaluating semantic intrusion errors to distinguish between amyloid positive and negative groups on the Alzheimer's disease continuum. *Journal of Psychiatric Research*. 2020; 124: 131–36.

Curiel Cid, RE, Crocco, EA, Duara, R, et al. Different aspects of failing to recover from proactive semantic interference predict rate of progression from amnestic mild cognitive impairment to dementia. *Frontiers in Aging Neuroscience*. 2024; 16: 1336008.

Curiel Cid, RE, Crocco, E, , Kitaigorodsky, M, et al.. A novel computerized cognitive stress test to detect mild cognitive impairment. *The Journal of Prevention of Alzheimer's Disease*. 2021; 8: 135–41.

Curiel, RE, Crocco, E, Acevedo, A, et al. A new scale for the evaluation of proactive and retroactive interference in mild cognitive impairment and early Alzheimer's disease. *Aging*. 2013; 1: 1000102.

Curiel, RE, Loewenstein, DA, Rosselli, M, et al. Semantic intrusions and failure to recover from semantic interference in mild cognitive impairment: Relationship to amyloid and cortical thickness. *Current Alzheimer Research*. 2018; 15: 848–55.

Cuschnir, C, Faiman, C. Adaptación y baremación para niños de la Prueba Visomotora de Bender. Editorial Paidos, Buenos Aires, Argentina: 1979.

Custodio, N, Lira, D, Montesinos, R, et al. [Usefulness of the Addenbrooke's Cognitive Examination (Spanish version) in Peruvian patients with Alzheimer's disease and Frontotemporal Dementia]. *Vertex*. 2012; 23: 165–72.

Custodio, N, Montesinos, R, Chambergo-Michilot, D, et al. A functional assessment tool to distinguish controls from Alzheimer's disease in Lima, Peru. *American Journal of Alzheimer's Disease and Other Dementias*. 2022; 37: 15333175221104354.

De la Torre, GG, Suarez-Llorens, A, Caballero, FJ, et al. Norms and reliability for the Spanish version of the Repeatable Battery for the Assessment of Neuropsychological Status (RBANS) Form A. *Journal of Clinical and Experimental Neuropsychology*. 2014; 36: 1023–30.

De las Cuevas, C, González de Rivera, JL, Henry-Benítez, M, et al. Análisis factorial de la versión española del SCL-90-R en la población general. *Anales de Psiquiatría*, 1991; 7: 93–96.

De Renzi, E, Vignolo, LA. The Token Test: A sensitive test to detect receptive disturbances in aphasics. *Brain: A Journal of Neurology*. 1962; 85: 665–78.

Del Pino, R, Peña, JN, Ibarretxe-Bilbao, N, et al. Demographically calibrated norms for two premorbid intelligence measures: The Word Accentuation Test and Pseudo-Words Reading subtest. *Frontiers in Psychology*. 2018; 9: 1950.

Del Ser, T, Gonzalez-Montalvo, JI, Martinez-Espinosa, S, et al. Estimation of premorbid intelligence in Spanish people with the Word Accentuation Test and its application to the diagnosis of dementia. *Brain and Cognition*. 1997; 33: 343–56.

Delgado, C, Araneda, A, Behrens, MI. Validation of the Spanish-language version of the Montreal Cognitive Assessment test in adults older than 60 years. *Neurología (English Edition)*. 2019; 34: 376–85.

Derogatis, LR, Yevzeroff, H, Wittelsberger, B. Social class, psychological disorder, and the nature of the psychopathologic indicator. *Journal of Consulting and Clinical Psychology*. 1975; 43: 183–91.

Díaz-Santos, M, Suárez, PA, Marquine, MJ, et al. Updated demographically adjusted norms for the Brief Visuospatial Memory Test-revised and Hopkins Verbal Learning Test-revised in Spanish-speakers from the U.S.-Mexico border region: The NP-NUMBRS project. *The Clinical Neuropsychologist*. 2020; 35: 374–95.

Duggan, EC, Awakon, LM, Loaiza, CC, et al. Contributing towards a cultural neuropsychology assessment decision-making framework: Comparison of WAIS-IV norms from Colombia, Chile, Mexico, Spain, United States, and Canada. *Archives of Clinical Neuropsychology*. 2019; 34: 657–81.

Dunn, AL, Fox Tree, JE. A quick, gradient Bilingual Dominance Scale. *Bilingualism: Language and Cognition*. 2009; 12: 273–89.

Escobedo, PS, Hollingworth, L. Annotations on the use of the Mexican norms for the WAIS-III. *Applied Neuropsychology*. 2009; 16: 223–7.

Espitia, A, Duarte, L. Neuronorma Colombia: Contributions and methodological characteristics. *Neurología (English Edition)*. 2024; 39: 10–19.

Farias, ST, Mungas, D, Reed, BR, et al. The measurement of everyday cognition (ECog): Scale development and psychometric properties. *Neuropsychology*. 2008; 22: 531–44.

Fernandez, AL. Modern neuropsychological tests for a diversity of cultural contexts. *The Clinical Neuropsychologist*. 2019; 33: 438–45.

Fernández-Blázquez, MA, Ávila-Villanueva, M, López-Pina, JA, et al. Psychometric properties of a new short version of the State-Trait Anxiety Inventory (STAI) for the assessment of anxiety in the elderly. *Neurología (English Edition)*. 2015; 30(6), 352-358.

Fernandez-San Martin, M, Andrade-Rosa, C, Molina, JD, et al. Validation of the Spanish version of the geriatric depression scale (GDS) in primary care. *International Journal of Geriatric Psychiatry*. 2002; 17: 279–87.

Field, A. *Discovering statistics using IBM SPSS statistics.* Sage Publications Limited: 2024.

Fillenbaum, GG, Kuchibhatla, M, Henderson, VM, et al. Comparison of performance on the CERAD neuropsychological battery of Hispanic patients and cognitively normal controls at two sites. *Clinical Gerontologist: The Journal of Aging and Mental Health*. 2007; 30: 1–22.

Folstein, MF, Folstein, SE, McHugh, PR. "Mini-mental state". A practical method for grading the cognitive state of patients for the clinician. *Journal of Psychiatric Research*. 1975; 12: 189–98.

Funes, CM, Hernandez Rodriguez, J, Lopez, SR. Norm comparisons of the Spanish-language and English-language WAIS-III: Implications for clinical assessment and test adaptation. *Psychological Assessment*. 2016; 28: 1709–15.

Galasko, D, Bennett, D, Sano, M, et al. An inventory to assess activities of daily living for clinical trials in Alzheimer's disease. The Alzheimer's Disease Cooperative Study. *Alzheimer Disease and Associated Disorders*. 1997; 11 Suppl 2: S33–9.

Galasko, D, Schmitt, F, Thomas, R, et al. Detailed assessment of activities of daily living in moderate to severe Alzheimer's disease. *Journal of the International Neuropsychological Society*. 2005; 11: 446–53.

Garcia-Campayo, J, Zamorano, E, Ruiz, MA, et al. Cultural adaptation into Spanish of the generalized anxiety disorder-7 (GAD-7) scale as a screening tool. *Health Quality Life Outcomes*. 2010; 8: 8.

Gasquoine, PG, Croyle, KL, Cavazos-Gonzalez, C, et al. Language of administration and neuropsychological test performance in neurologically intact Hispanic American bilingual adults. *Archives of Clinical Neuropsychology*. 2007; 22: 991–1001.

Gershon, RC, Fox, RS, Manly, JJ, et al. The NIH Toolbox: Overview of development for use with Hispanic populations. *Journal of the International Neuropsychological Society*. 2020; 26: 567–75.

Gleichgerrcht, E, Camino, J, Roca, M, et al. Assessment of functional impairment in dementia with the Spanish version of the Activities of Daily Living Questionnaire. *Dementia and Geriatric Cognitive Disorders*. 2009; 28: 380–8.

Golden, C, Freshwater, SM, Golden, Z. Stroop color and word test. Wood Dale, Illinois Stoelting Company: 1978.

Gollan, TH, Weissberger, GH, Runnqvist, E, et al. Self-ratings of spoken language dominance: A Multilingual Naming Test (MINT) and preliminary norms for young and aging Spanish–English bilinguals. *Bilingualism: Language and Cognition*. 2012; 15: 594–615.

Gonzalez, DA, Gonzales, MM, Resch, ZJ, et al. Comprehensive evaluation of the Functional Activities Questionnaire (FAQ) and its reliability and validity. *Assessment*. 2022; 29: 748–63.

González de Rivera, JL, Derogatis, LR, De las Cuevas, C, et al. The Spanish version of the SCL-90-R. Normative data in the general population. *Towson: Clinical Psychometric Research*. 1989.

Gonzalez, HM, Tarraf, W, Gonzalez, KA, et al. Diabetes, Cognitive Decline, and Mild Cognitive Impairment Among Diverse Hispanics/Latinos: Study of Latinos-Investigation of Neurocognitive Aging Results (HCHS/SOL). *Diabetes Care*, 2020; 43: 1111–17.

González, HM, Mungas, D, Haan, MN. A verbal learning and memory test for English- and Spanish-speaking older Mexican-American adults. *The Clinical Neuropsychologist*, 2002; 16: 439–51.

González, HM, Mungas, D, Reed, BR, et al. A new verbal learning and memory test for English-and Spanish-speaking older people. *Journal of the International Neuropsychological Society*. 2001; 7: 544–55.

González Ordi, H, Santamaría Fernández, P. *Adaptación Española del Inventario Estructurado de Simulación de Síntomas – SIMS*. TEA Ediciones, Madrid, Spain: 2009.

Goodglass, H, Kaplan, E. The *Assessment of Aphasia and Related Disorders* (2nd ed.). Lea & Febiger: Philadelphia, PA, U.S.: 1983.

Goodglass, H, Kaplan, E, Barresi, B. *The Assessment of Aphasia and Related Disorders* (3rd ed.). Lippincott Williams & Wilkins: Philadelphia, PA, U.S.: 2001.

Goodman, ZT, Llabre, MM, Gonzalez, HM, et al. Testing measurement equivalence of neurocognitive assessments across language in the Hispanic Community Health Study/Study of Latinos. *Neuropsychology*. 2021; 35: 423–33.

Gouveia, PAR, Brucki, SMD, Malheiros, SMF, et al. Disorders in planning and strategy application in frontal lobe lesion patients. *Brain and Cognition*. 2007; 63: 240–46.

Grant, DA, and Berg, EA. *Wisconsin Card Sorting Test.* APA Psycnet, Washington, DC, U.S.: 2014.

Grober, E, Sanders, AE, Hall, C, et al. Free and cued selective reminding identifies very mild dementia in primary care. *Alzheimer Disease and Associated Disorders*. 2010; 24: 284–90.

Guardia-Olmos, J, Pero-Cebollero, M, Rivera, D, et al. Methodology for the development of normative data for ten Spanish-language neuropsychological tests in eleven Latin American countries. *NeuroRehabilitation*. 2015; 37: 493–9.

Guerrero-Berroa, E, Schmeidler, J, Raventos, H, et al. Neuropsychological test performance in cognitively normal Spanish-speaking nonagenarians with little education. *Journal of Cross-Cultural Gerontology*. 2016; 31: 129–41.

Hall, JR, Balldin, VH, Gamboa, A, et al. Texas Mexican American adult normative studies: Normative data for the Repeatable Battery for the Assessment of Neuropsychological Status (RBANS). *Developmental Neuropsychology*. 2018; 43: 27–35.

Harvey, P, Curiel-Cid, R, Kallestrup, P, et al. Digital migration of the Loewenstein Acevedo Scales for Semantic Interference and Learning (LASSI-L): Development and validation study in older participants. *JMIR Mental Health*. 2025; 12: e64716.

Heaton, A, Gooding, A, Cherner, M, et al. Demographically-adjusted norms for the Grooved Pegboard and Finger Tapping tests in Spanish-speaking adults: Results from the Neuropsychological Norms for the U.S.-Mexico Border Region in Spanish (NP-NUMBRS) Project. *The Clinical Neuropsychologist*. 2021; 35: 396–418.

Heaton, RK, Chelune, GJ, Talley, JL, et al. Wisconsin Card Sorting Test Manual (4th ed.). Psychological Assessment Resources: Odessa, FL, U.S.: 1993.

Heaton, RK, Grant, I Matthews, CG. *Comprehensive Norms for an Expanded Halstead-Reitan Battery: Demographic Corrections, Research Findings, and Clinical Applications.* Psychological Assessment Resources, Inc., Odessa, FL, U.S.: 1991.

Henao-Arboleda, E, Muñoz, C, Aguirre-Acevedo, DC, et al. Datos normativos de pruebas neuropsicológicas en adultos mayores en una población Colombiana. *Revista Chilena de Neuropsicología*. 2010; 5: 214–26.

Henrich, J, Heine, SJ, and Norenzayan, A. The weirdest people in the world?. *The Behavioral and Brain Sciences*. 2010; 33: 61–83; discussion 83–135.

Inesta, C, Oltra-Cucarella, J, Bonete-Lopez, B, et al. Regression-based normative data for independent and cognitively active Spanish older adults: Digit Span, Letters and Numbers, Trail Making Test and Symbol Digit Modalities Test. *International Journal of Environmental Research and Public Health*. 2021; 18: 9958

Ismail, Z, Elbayoumi, H, Fischer, CE, et al. Prevalence of depression in patients with mild cognitive impairment: A systematic review and meta-analysis. *JAMA Psychiatry*. 2017; 74: 58–67.

Jacobs, J. Experiments on "prehension". *Mind*. 1887; 12: 75–79.

Jahn, DR, Mauer, CB, Menon, CV, et al. A brief Spanish-English equivalent version of the Boston Naming Test: A Project FRONTIER study. *Journal of Clinical and Experimental Neuropsychology*. 2013; 35: 835–45.

Johnson, N, Barion, A, Rademaker, A, et al. The Activities of Daily Living Questionnaire: A validation study in patients with dementia. *Alzheimer's Disease & Associated Disorders*. 2004; 18: 223–30.

Julayanont, P, and DeToledo, JC. Validity of the Clinical Dementia Rating Scale Sum of Boxes in staging and detection of cognitive impairment in Mexican Americans. *Journal of Geriatric Psychiatry and Neurology*. 2022; 35: 128–34.

Julio-Ramos, T, Mora-Castelletto, V, Conejeros-Pavez, J, et al. Validation of the abbreviated version of the Token Test in Latin American Spanish stroke patients. *International Journal of Language & Communication Disorders*. 2024; 59: 2815–27.

Jurica, PJ, Leitten, CL, and Mattis, S. Dementia Rating Scale-2 (DRS-2): *Professional Manual. Psychological Assessment Resources*. Odessa, FL, U.S.: 2001.

Kaplan, E, Goodglass, H, Weintraub, S. *Boston Naming Test: An Experimental Version.* Boston VA Medical Center: Boston, MA, U.S.: 1998.

Kessels, RPM, van Zandvoort, J, Postma, A, et al. *The Corsi block-tapping task: Standardization and normative data. Applied Neuropsychology*. 2000; 7: 252–8.

Klove, H. Clinical Neuropsychology. *The Medical Clinics of North America*. 1963; 47: 1647–58.

Kobylecki, C, Jones, M, Thompson, JC, et al. Cognitive-behavioural features of progressive supranuclear palsy syndrome overlap with frontotemporal dementia. *Journal of Neurology*. 2015; 262: 916–22.

Kramer, JH, Jurik, J, Sha, SJ, et al. Distinctive neuropsychological patterns in frontotemporal dementia, semantic dementia, and Alzheimer disease. *Cognitive and Behavioral Neurology*. 2003; 16: 211–8.

Kreutzer, JS, DeLuca, J, and Caplan, B. *Encyclopedia of Clinical Neuropsychology*. Springer, New York, NY: 2018.

Kroenke, K, Spitzer, RL, and Williams, JB. The PHQ-9: Validity of a brief depression severity measure. *Journal of General Internal Medicine*. 2001; 16: 606–13.

Labos, E, Trojanowski, S, and Ruiz, C. Prueba de recuerdo libre/facilitado con recuerdo inmediato. Versión verbal de la FCSRT-IR. Adaptación y normas en lengua española. *Revista Neurológica Argentina*. 2008; 33: 50–66.

LaForte, EM, Wendling, BJ, Mather, N, et al. *Batería IV Woodcock-Muñoz Technical Abstract (Batería IV Assessment Service Bulletin No. 1)*. Riverside Insights, Itasca, IL: 2019.

Lamar, M, Glover, CM, Capuano, AW, et al. Stability and change in acculturation-related characteristics in older Latinos: Implications for culturally compatible ADRD research. *Alzheimer's & Dementia (N Y)*. 2023; 9: e12380.

Lansing, AE, Ivnik, RJ, Cullum, CM, et al. An empirically derived short form of the Boston Naming Test. *Archives of Clinical Neuropsychology*. 1999; 14: 481–7.

Lezak, MD, Howieson, DB, Bigler, ED, et al. *Neuropsychological Assessment*. Oxford University Press, Oxford, England: 2012 .

Li, P, Sepanski, S, and Zhao, X. Language history questionnaire: A web-based interface for bilingual research. *Behavior Research Methods*. 2006; 38: 202–10.

Li, P, Zhang, F, Yu, A, et al. Language History Questionnaire (LHQ3): An enhanced tool for assessing multilingual experience. *Bilingualism: Language and Cognition*. 2020; 23: 938–44.

Loewenstein, DA, Argüelles, T, Argüelles, S, et al. Potential cultural bias in the neuropsychological assessment of the older adult. *Journal of Clinical and Experimental Neuropsychology*. 1994; 16: 623–29.

Loewenstein, DA, Curiel, RE, Greig, MT, et al. A novel cognitive stress test for the detection of preclinical Alzheimer Disease: Discriminative properties and relation to amyloid load. *The American Journal of Geriatric Psychiatry*. 2016; 24: 804–13.

Loewenstein, DA, Curiel, RE, Wright, C, et al. Recovery from Proactive Semantic Interference in Mild Cognitive Impairment and Normal Aging: Relationship to Atrophy in Brain Regions Vulnerable to Alzheimer's Disease. *Journal of Alzheimer's Disease*. 2017; 56: 1119–26.

Lucas-Carrasco, R. Spanish version of the Geriatric Depression Scale: Reliability and validity in persons with mild-moderate dementia. *International Psychogeriatrics*. 2012; 24: 1284–90.

Magan, I, Sanz, J, Garcia-Vera, MP. Psychometric properties of a Spanish version of the Beck Anxiety Inventory (BAI) in general population. *The Spanish Journal of Psychology*. 2008; 11: 626–40.

Maj, M, D'Elia, L, Satz, P, et al. Evaluation of two new neuropsychological tests designed to minimize cultural bias in the assessment of HIV-1 seropositive persons: A WHO study. *Archives of Clinical Neuropsychology*. 1993; 8: 123–35.

Malcarne, VL, Chavira, DA, Fernandez, S, et al. The Scale of Ethnic Experience: Development and psychometric properties. *Journal of Personality Assessment*. 2006; 86: 150–61.

Mallo, SC, Ismail, Z, Pereiro, AX, et al. Assessing mild behavioral impairment with the Mild Behavioral Impairment-Checklist in people with mild cognitive impairment. *Journal of Alzheimer's Disease*. 2018; 66: 83–95.

Manly, JJ, Jacobs, DM, Touradji, P, et al. Reading level attenuates differences in neuropsychological test performance between African American and White elders. *Journal of the International Neuropsychological Society*. 2002; 8: 341–8.

Marian, V, Blumenfeld, HK, and Kaushanskaya, M. The Language Experience and Proficiency Questionnaire (LEAP-Q): Assessing language profiles in bilinguals and multilinguals. *Journal of Speech, Language, and Hearing Research*. 2007; 50: 940–67.

Marin, G, and Gamba, RJ. A new measurement of acculturation for Hispanics: The Bidimensional Acculturation Scale for Hispanics (BAS). *Hispanic Journal of Behavioral Sciences*. 1996; 18: 297–316.

Marín, G, Sabogal, F, Marín, BV, et al. Development of a short acculturation scale for Hispanics. *Hispanic Journal of Behavioral Sciences*. 1987; 9: 183–205.

Marks, RA, Labotka, D, Sun, X, et al. Morphological awareness and its role in early word reading in English monolinguals, Spanish-English, and Chinese-English simultaneous bilinguals. *Bilingualism (Cambridge, England)*. 2023; 26: 268–83.

Marquez de la Plata, C, Vicioso, B, Hynan, L, et al. Development of the Texas Spanish Naming Test: Atest for Spanish speakers. *The Clinical Neuropsychologist*. 2008; 22: 288–304.

Marquez de la Plata, C, Arango-Lasprilla, JC, Alegret, M, et al. Item analysis of three Spanish naming tests: A cross-cultural investigation. *NeuroRehabilitation*. 2009; 24: 75–85.

Marquez-Gonzalez, M, Losada, A, Fernandez-Fernandez, V, et al. Psychometric properties of the Spanish version of the Geriatric Anxiety Inventory. *International Psychogeriatrics*. 2012; 24: 137–44.

Marquine, MJ, Morlett Paredes, A, Madriaga, C, et al. Demographically-adjusted norms for selected tests of verbal fluency: Results from the Neuropsychological Norms for the U.S.-Mexico Border Region in Spanish (NP-NUMBRS) project. *The Clinical Neuropsychologist*. 2021; 35: 269–92.

Marquine, MJ, Parks, A, Perales-Puchalt, J, et al. Demographically-adjusted normative data among Latinos for the version 3 of the Alzheimer's Disease Centers' Neuropsychological Test Battery in the Uniform Data Set. *Alzheimer's & Dementia*. 2023; 19: 4174–86.

Marquine, MJ, Yassai-Gonzalez, D, Perez-Tejada, A, et al. Demographically adjusted normative data for the Wisconsin Card Sorting Test-64 item: Results from the Neuropsychological Norms for the U.S.–Mexico Border Region in Spanish (NP-NUMBRS) project. *The Clinical Neuropsychologist*. 2021; 35: 339–55.

Martínez de la Iglesia, J, Onís Vilches, M, Dueñas Herrero, R, et al. Versión española del cuestionario de Yesavage abreviado (GDS) para el despistaje de depresión en mayores de 65 años: Adaptación y validación. *Medifam*. 2002; 12: 26–40.

Matias-Guiu, JA, Cortes-Martinez, A, Valles-Salgado, M, et al. Addenbrooke's cognitive examination III: Diagnostic utility for mild cognitive impairment and dementia and correlation with standardized neuropsychological tests. *International Psychogeriatrics*, 2017; 29: 105-13.

Matias-Guiu, JA, Fernandez de Bobadilla, R, Escudero, G, et al. Validation of the Spanish version of Addenbrooke's Cognitive Examination III for diagnosing dementia. *Neurología*. 2015; 30: 545–51.

Matthews, KA, Hall, MH, Lee, L, et al. Racial/ethnic disparities in women's sleep duration, continuity, and quality, and their statistical mediators: Study of Women's Health Across the Nation. *Sleep*. 2019; 42.

McGrew, KS, Schneider, WJ, Decker, SL, et al. A psychometric network analysis of CHC intelligence measures: Implications for research, theory, and interpretation of broad CHC Scores "Beyond g". *Journal of Intelligence*. 2023;11 (1), 19.

Mendoza, L, Garcia, P, Padron, D, et al. Reliability and validity of the MCDR for Hispanic older adults. *Innovation in Aging*. 2023; 7: 596.

Merckelbach, H, Smith, GP. Diagnostic accuracy of the Structured Inventory of Malingered Symptomatology (SIMS) in detecting instructed malingering. *Archives of Clinical Neuropsychology*. 2003;18: 145–52.

Merz, EL, Malcarne, VL, Roesch, SC, et al. A multigroup confirmatory factor analysis of the Patient Health Questionnaire-9 among English- and Spanish-speaking Latinas. *Cultural Diversity & Ethnic Minority Psychology*. 2011; 17: 309–16.

Meyers, JE, and Meyers, KR. Rey Complex Figure Test under four different administration procedures. *The Clinical Neuropsychologist*. 1995; 9: 63–67.

Miller, GA. The magical number seven, plus or minus two: Some limits on our capacity for processing information. *Psychological Review*. 1956; 63: 81–97.

Mills, SD, Fox, RS, Malcarne, VL, et al. The psychometric properties of the generalized anxiety disorder-7 scale in Hispanic Americans with English or Spanish language preference. *Cultural Diversity & Ethnic Minority Psychology*. 2014; 20: 463–68.

Mokri, H, Avila-Funes, JA, Meillon, C, et al. Normative data for the Mini-Mental State Examination, the Free and Cued Selective Reminding Test and the Isaacs Set Test for an older adult Mexican population: The Coyoacan cohort study. *The Clinical Neuropsychologist*. 2013; 27: 1004–18.

Montañes, P, Espitia, A, d Duarte L. *Neuronorma Colombia: Protocolo, Normas, Plataforma de Perfiles Neuropsicológicos y Aplicaciones Clínicas.* Universidad Nacional de Colombia, Bogotá, Colombia: 2020.

Morales, M, Campo, P, Fernández, A, et al. Normative data for a six-trial administration of a Spanish version of the Verbal Selective Reminding Test. *Archives of Clinical Neuropsychology*. 2010; 25: 745–61.

Morel Valdes, GM, Rivera, D, Olabarrieta-Landa, L, et al. Normative data for tests of visuo-spatial, visuo-constructional skills, and visual memory for Spanish-speaking adults in the United States. *NeuroRehabilitation*. 2024; 55: 223–33.

Morlett Paredes, A, Gooding, A, Fortuny L. Artiola, I, et al. The state of neuropsychological test norms for Spanish-speaking adults in the United States. *The Clinical Neuropsychologist*. 2021; 35: 236–52.

Morris, JC, Mohs, RC, Rogers, H, et al. Consortium to establish a registry for Alzheimer's disease (CERAD) clinical and neuropsychological assessment of Alzheimer's disease. *Psychopharmacology Bulletin*. 1988; 24: 641–52.

Mungas, D, Reed, BR, Crane, PK, et al. Spanish and English Neuropsychological Assessment Scales (SENAS): Further development and psychometric characteristics. *Psychological Assessment*. 2004; 16: 347–59.

Muñoz-Neira, C, Lopez, OL, Riveros, R, et al. The technology – activities of daily living questionnaire: A version with a technology-related subscale. *Dementia and Geriatric Cognitive Disorders*. 2012; 33: 361–71.

Muñoz-Sandoval, AF, Woodcock, RW, McGrew, KS, et al. *Batería III Pruebas de Aprovechamiento.* Riverside Publishing, Itasca, IL, U.S.: 2005.

Muntal Encinas, S, Gramunt-Fombuena, N, Badenes Guia, D, et al. Spanish translation and adaptation of the repeatable battery for the assessment of neuropsychological status (RBANS) Form A in a pilot sample. *Neurología*. 2012; 27: 531–46.

Muntal, S, Doval, E, Badenes, D, et al. New normative data from the Spanish-language version of the Repeatable Battery for the Assessment of Neuropsychological Status (RBANS), form A. *Neurología (English Edition)*. 2020; 35: 303–10.

Muroya, N, Inoue, T, Hosokawa, M, et al. The role of morphological awareness in word reading kills in Japanese: A within-language cross-orthographic perspective. *Scientific Studies of Reading*. 2017; 21: 449–62.

Musa, G, Henriquez, F, Munoz-Neira, C, et al. Utility of the Neuropsychiatric Inventory Questionnaire (NPI-Q) in the assessment of a sample of patients with Alzheimer's disease in Chile. *Dementia & Neuropsychologia*. 2017; 11: 129–36.

Nasreddine, ZS, Phillips, NA, Bedirian, V, et al. The Montreal Cognitive Assessment, MoCA: A brief screening tool for mild cognitive impairment. *Journal of the American Geriatrics Society*. 2005; 53: 695–9.

Nelson, HE. A modified card sorting test sensitive to frontal lobe defects. *Cortex*. 1976; 12: 313–24.

Nelson, HE, Willison, JR. *The revised National Adult Reading Test – Test manual.* NFER-Nelson, Windsor, UK: 1991.

O'Bryant, SE, Edwards, M, Johnson, L, et al. Texas Mexican American adult normative studies: Normative data for commonly used clinical neuropsychological measures for English- and Spanish-speakers. *Developmental Neuropsychology*. 2018; 43: 1–26.

Olabarrieta-Landa, L, Rivera, D, Morlett-Paredes, A, et al. Standard form of the Boston Naming Test: Normative data for the Latin American Spanish speaking adult population. *NeuroRehabilitation*. 2015; 37(4): 501–13.

Olabarrieta-Landa, L, Rivera, D, Xia, B, et al. Normative data for verbal fluency and naming tests in Spanish-speaking adults in the United States. *NeuroRehabilitation*. 2024; 55: 195–208.

Oquendo-Jimenez, I, Mena, R, Antoun, MD, et al. Linguistic adaptation of the Clinical Dementia Rating scale for a Spanish-speaking population: A focus group approach. *Puerto Rico Health Sciences Journal*. 2010; 29: 102–8.

Ordi, HG, Fernández, PS, and Marín, PF. Precisión predictiva del Inventario Estructurado de Simulación de Síntomas-SIMS en el contexto medicolegal [Predictive accuracy of the Structured Inventory of Malingered Symptomatology-SIMS in the medicolegal setting]. *EduPsykhé: Revista de Psicología y Educación*. 2010; 9: 3–22.

Osterrieth, PA. Le test de copie d'une figure complexe; contribution à l'étude de la perception et de la mémoire [Test of copying a complex figure; contribution to the study of perception and memory]. *Archives de Psychologie*. 1944; 30: 206–356.

Ostrosky-Solis, F, Ardila, A, Rosselli, M. NEUROPSI: A brief neuropsychological test battery in Spanish with norms by age and educational level. *Journal of the International Neuropsychological Society*. 1999; 5: 413–33.

Ostrosky-Solis, F, Ardila, A, Rosselli, M, et al. Neuropsychological test performance in illiterate subjects. *Archives of Clinical Neuropsychology*. 1998; 13: 645–60.

Ostrosky-Solis, F, Gomez-Perez, ME, Matute, E, et al. NEUROPSI Attention and Memory: A neuropsychological test battery in Spanish with norms by age and educational level. *Applied Neuropsychology*. 2007; 14: 156–70.

Ostrosky-Solis, F, Lopez-Arango, G, a Ardila, A. Sensitivity and specificity of the Mini-Mental State Examination in a Spanish-speaking population. *Applied Neuropsychology*. 2000; 7: 25–31.

Pagán-Torres, OM, Cumba-Avilés, E, Rosario-Hernández, E, et al. Reviewing the Psychometric Properties and Factor Structure of the Generalized Anxiety Disorder-7 (GAD-7) in a Sample of Puerto Rican Adults. *International Journal of Recent Scientific Research*. 2020; 11: 36885–88.

Palomo, R, Casals-Coll, M, Sanchez-Benavides, G, et al. Spanish normative studies in young adults (NEURONORMA young adults project): Norms for the Rey-Osterrieth Complex Figure (copy and memory) and Free and Cued Selective Reminding Test. *Neurología*. 2013; 28: 226–35.

Peña-Casanova, J, Blesa, R, Aguilar, M, et al. Spanish Multicenter Normative Studies (NEURONORMA Project): Methods and sample characteristics. *Archives of Clinical Neuropsychology*. 2009; 24: 307–19.

Peña-Casanova, J, Casals-Coll, M, Quintana, M, et al. [Spanish normative studies in a young adult population (NEURONORMA young adults Project): Methods and characteristics of the sample]. *Neurología*. 2012; 27: 253–60.

Peña-Casanova, J, Gramunt-Fombuena, N, Quinones-Ubeda, S, et al. Spanish Multicenter Normative Studies (NEURONORMA Project): Norms for the Rey-Osterrieth complex figure (copy and memory), and free and cued selective reminding test. *Archives of Clinical Neuropsychology*. 2009; 24: 371–93.

Peña-Casanova, J, Quinones-Ubeda, S, Gramunt-Fombuena, N, et al. Spanish Multicenter Normative Studies (NEURONORMA Project): Norms for Boston naming test and token test. *Archives of Clinical Neuropsychology*. 2009; 24: 343–54.

Peña-Casanova, J, Quinones-Ubeda, S, Quintana-Aparicio, M, et al. Spanish Multicenter Normative Studies (NEURONORMA Project): Norms for verbal span, visuospatial span, letter and number sequencing, trail making test, and symbol digit modalities test. *Archives of Clinical Neuropsychology*. 2009; 24: 321–41.

Peña-Casanova, J, Quintana-Aparicio, M, Quinones-Ubeda, S, et al. Spanish Multicenter Normative Studies (NEURONORMA Project): Norms for the visual object and space perception battery-abbreviated, and judgment of line orientation. *Archives of Clinical Neuropsychology*. 2009; 24: 355–70.

Penley, JA, Wiebe, JS, and Nwosu, A. Psychometric properties of the Spanish Beck Depression Inventory-II in a medical sample. *Psychological Assessment*. 2003;15: 569–77.

Pereiro, AX, Ramos-Lema, S, Lojo-Seoane, C, et al. Normative data for the Montreal Cognitive Assessment (MOCA) in a Spanish sample of community-dweller adults. *European Geriatric Medicine*. 2017; 8: 240–44.

Perez-Lao, A, Ying, G, Arias, F, et al. A systematic review of available normative data on neuropsychological tests for Spanish speakers in the U.S., Latin America and the Caribbean, and Spain. *Neuropsychology Review*. 2025; 35(3), 451–478.

Petersen, RC, Smith, G, Kokmen, E, et al. Memory function in normal aging. *Neurology*. 1992; 42: 396–401.

Pfeffer, RI, Kurosaki, TT, Harrah Jr., CH, et al. Measurement of functional activities in older adults in the community. *Journal of Gerontology*. 1982; 37: 323–9.

Phinney, JS. The multigroup ethnic identity measure: A new scale for use with diverse groups. *Journal of Adolescent Research*. 1992; 72: 156–76.

Pineda, DA, Rosselli, M, Ardila, A, et al. The Boston Diagnostic Aphasia Examination-Spanish version: The influence of demographic variables. *Journal of the International Neuropsychological Society*. 2000; 6: 802–14.

Pons, JI, Flores-Pabón, L, Matías-Carrelo, L, et al. Confiabilidad de la Escala de Inteligencia Wechsler para Adultos Versión III, Puerto Rico (EIWA-III) [Reliability of the Wechsler Adult Intelligence Scale Version III, Puerto Rico (EIWA-III)]. *Revista Puertorriqueña de Psicología*. 2008; 19: 112–32.

Ponton, MO, Satz, P, Herrera, L, et al. Normative data stratified by age and education for the Neuropsychological Screening Battery for Hispanics (NeSBHIS): Initial report. *Journal of the International Neuropsychological Society*. 1996; 2: 96–104.

Potashman, M, Pang, M, Tahir, M, et al. Psychometric properties of the Alzheimer's Disease Cooperative Study – Activities of Daily Living for Mild Cognitive Impairment (ADCS-MCI-ADL) scale: A post hoc analysis of the ADCS ADC-008 trial. *BMC Geriatrics*. 2023; 23: 124.

Prins, ND, van Dijk, EJ, den Heijer, T, et al. Cerebral small-vessel disease and decline in information processing speed, executive function and memory. *Brain*. 2005; 128: 2034–41.

Querejeta, AN, Farías, Y, Moreno, MA, et al. Test Neuropsi: Normas según edad y nivel de instrucción para Argentina. *Cuadernos de Neuropsicología*. 2012; 6: 153–64.

Quiroz, YT, Solis, M, Aranda, MP, et al. Addressing the disparities in dementia risk, early detection and care in Latino populations: Highlights from the second Latinos & Alzheimer's Symposium. *Alzheimer's & Dementia*. 2022; 18: 1677–86.

Ramos Usuga, D, Ayearst, LE, Rivera, D, et al. A preliminary examination of the TOMM2 in a sample of Spanish speakers in the United States. *NeuroRehabilitation*. 2024; 55: 235–42.

Ramos Usuga, D, Rivera, D, Xia, B, et al. Executive function tests: Normative data for Spanish-speaking adults in the United States. *NeuroRehabilitation*. 2024; 55: 209–21.

Randolph, C, Tierney, MC, Mohr, E, et al. The Repeatable Battery for the Assessment of Neuropsychological Status (RBANS): Preliminary clinical validity. *Journal of Clinical and Experimental Neuropsychology*. 1998; 20: 310–9.

Rankin, KP, Toller, G, Gavron, L, et al. Social Behavior Observer Checklist: Patterns of Spontaneous Behaviors Differentiate Patients With Neurodegenerative Disease From Healthy Older Adults. *Frontiers in Neurology*. 2021; 12: 683162.

Rascovsky, K. A primer in neuropsychological assessment for dementia. *Practical Neurology*. 2016; 15: 20–25.

Raven, J. The Raven's progressive matrices: Change and stability over culture and time. *Cognitive Psychology*. 2000; 41: 1–48.

Raven, JC. R*aven's 2, Matrices Progresivas de Raven*|Segunda edición, *Spain Version: Manual para la Administración, Corrección e Interpretación*. Pearson Clinical and Talent Assessment, San Antonio, TX, U.S.: 2019.

Raven, JC. *Coloured Progressive Matrices Sets A, Ab, B. Manual Sections 1 & 2*. Oxford Psychologists Press, Oxford, UK: 1995

Raven, JC. *Progressive Matrices: A Perceptual Test of Intelligence*. Lewis Raven, London, UK: 1938.

Reitan, RM. Validity of the Trail Making Test as an indicator of organic brain damage. *Perceptual and Motor Skills*. 1958; 8: 271–76.

Reitan, RM, and Wolfson, D. *The Halstead–Reitan Neuropsychological Test Battery: Therapy and Clinical Interpretation*. Neuropsychological Press: Tucson, AZ: 1985.

Renteria, L, Li, ST, and Pliskin, NH. Reliability and validity of the Spanish Language Wechsler Adult Intelligence Scale (3rd Edition) in a sample of American, urban, Spanish-speaking Hispanics. *The Clinical Neuropsychologist*. 2008; 22: 455–70.

Rey, A, and Osterrieth, PA. Rey-Osterrieth Complex Figure Copying Test [Database record]. APA PsycTests, Washington D.C.: 1941.

Rey, G and Benton, A. Exámen de Afasia Multilingüe (Multilingual Aphasia Examination-Spanish). AJA Associates, Inc., Iowa City, Iowa: 1991.

Rey, GJ, Feldman, E, Rivas-Vazquez, R, et al. Neuropsychological test development and normative data on Hispanics. *Archives of Clinical Neuropsychology*. 1999; 14: 593–601.

Reynolds, CR, and Kamphaus, RW. *RIAS: Escalas de Inteligencia de Reynolds*. TEA, Madrid, Spain: 2013.

Rivera, D, Forte, A, Olabarrieta-Landa, L, et al. Methodology for the generation of normative data for the U.S. adult Spanish-speaking population: A Bayesian approach. *NeuroRehabilitation*. 2024; 55: 155–67.

Rivera, D, Perrin, PB, Weiler, G, et al. Test of Memory Malingering (TOMM): Normative data for the Latin American Spanish speaking adult population. *NeuroRehabilitation*. 2015; 37: 719–35.

Rivera, D, Olabarrieta-Landa, L, Van der Elst, W, et al. Normative data for verbal fluency in healthy Latin American adults: Letter M, and fruits and occupations categories. *Neuropsychology*. 2019; 33: 287.

Rivera, D, Perrin, PB, Flores Stevens, L, et al. Stroop Color-Word Interference Test: Normative data for the Latin American Spanish speaking adult population. *NeuroRehabilitation*. 2015; 37: 591–624.

Rodriguez-Gomez, JR, Davila-Martinez, MG, and Collazo-Rodriguez, LC. Factor structure of the Beck Depression Inventory-Second Edition (BDI-II) with Puerto Rican elderly. *Puerto Rico Health Sciences Journal*. 2006; 25: 127–32.

Rodríguez-Lorenzana, A, Benito-Sánchez, I, Adana-Díaz, L, et al. Normative data for test of verbal fluency and naming on Ecuadorian adult population. *Frontiers in Psychology*. 2020; 11: 830.

Romero Vanegas, SJ, Valencia Marín, CM, Aguirre Acevedo, DC, et al. Alteraciones de la memoria episódica verbal en fases preclínica y temprana de la enfermedad de Alzheimer familiar precoz por mutaciónE280A en PS1. *Acta Neurológica Colombiana*. 2010; 26: 177–94.

Rosario-Hernandez, E, Rovira-Millan, LV, Merino-Soto, C, et al. Review of the psychometric properties of the Patient Health Questionnaire-9 (PHQ-9) Spanish version in a sample of Puerto Rican workers. *Frontiers in Psychiatry*. 2023; 14: 1024676.

Rosas, R, Tenorio, M, Pizarro, M, et al. Estandarización de la Escala Wechsler de Inteligencia para adultos-Cuarta Edición en Chile. *Psykhe (Santiago)*. 2014; 23: 1–18.

Rosen, WG, Terry, RD, Fuld, PA, et al. Pathological verification of ischemic score in differentiation of dementias. *Annals of Neurology*. 1980; 7: 486–8.

Rosselli, D, Ardila, A, Pradilla, G, et al. [The Mini-Mental State Examination as a selected diagnostic test for dementia: A Colombian population study. GENECO]. *Revista de Neurología*. 2000; 30: 428–32.

Rosselli, M, Ardila, A, Florez, A, et al. Normative data on the Boston Diagnostic Aphasia Examination in a Spanish-speaking population. *Journal of Clinical and Experimental Neuropsychology*. 1990; 12: 313–22.

Royall, DR, Mahurin, RK, and Gray, KF. Bedside assessment of executive cognitive impairment: The executive interview. *Journal of the American Geriatrics Society*. 1992; 40: 1221–6.

Ruff, RM, Light, RH, Parker,SB, et al. Benton controlled oral word association test: Reliability and updated norms. *Archives of Clinical Neuropsychology*. 1996; 11: 329–38.

Russo, MJ, Cohen, G, Chrem Mendez, P, et al. Utility of the Spanish version of the Everyday Cognition scale in the diagnosis of mild cognitive impairment and mild dementia in an older cohort from the Argentina-ADNI. *Aging Clinical and Experimental Research*. 2018; 30: 1167–76.

Ryan, J, Woods, RL, Britt, CJ, et al. Normative data for the Symbol Digit Modalities Test in older white Australians and Americans, African-Americans, and Hispanic/Latinos. *Journal of Alzheimer's Disease Reports*. 2020; 4: 313–23.

Sabogal, F, Marín, G, Otero-Sabogal, R, et al. Hispanic Familism and Acculturation: What Changes and What Doesn't?. *Hispanic Journal of Behavioral Sciences*. 1987; 9: 397–412.

Sáez-Atxukarro, O, Del Pino, R, Pena, J, et al. Hopkins Verbal Learning Test-revised: Normalization and standardization for Spanish population. *Revista de Neurología*. 2021; 72: 35–42.

Sanz, J, Perdigón, MA, and Vázquez, C. Adaptación española del Inventario para la Depresión de Beck-II (BDI-II): 2. Propiedades psicométricas en población general [Spanish adaptation of the Beck Depression Inventory-II (BDI-II): 2. Psychometric properties in the general population]. *Psicotema*. 2003; 15: 253–60.

Sanz-Morejón, A, Herrero-Fernández, D, Pacho-Pacho, DP, et al. Beck Anxiety Inventory: Psychometric characteristics in a sample from the clinical Spanish population. *Clinical & Health*. 2014; 25: 209–16.

Sawamoto, N, Honda, M, Hanakawa, T, et al. Cognitive slowing in Parkinson's disease: A behavioral evaluation independent of motor slowing. *Journal of Neuroscience*. 2002; 22: 5198–203.

Sayegh, P, and Knight, BG. Functional assessment and neuropsychiatric inventory questionnaires: Measurement invariance across Hispanics and non-Hispanic whites. *Gerontologist*. 2014; 54: 375–86.

Scarpina, F, and Tagini, S. The stroop color and word test. *Frontiers in Psychology*, 2017; 8: 557.

Schrauf, RW, Weintraub, S, Navarro, E. Is adaptation of the word accentuation test of premorbid intelligence necessary for use among older, Spanish-speaking immigrants in the United States?. *Journal of the International Neuropsychological Society*. 2006; 12: 391–9.

Schretlen, D. Brief Test of Attention professional manual. Psychological Assessment Resources, Odessa, FL, U.S.: 1997.

Scott, TM, Morlett Paredes, A, Taylor, MJ, et al. Demographically-adjusted norms for the WAIS-R Block Design and Arithmetic subtests: Results from the Neuropsychological Norms for the U.S.-Mexico Border Region in Spanish (NP-NUMBRS) project. *The Clinical Neuropsychologist*. 2021; 35: 419–32.

Sepanski, S, Li, P. Sentence processing in late bilinguals: Comprehension of form and meaning. *Journal of Cognitive Science*. 2007; 8: 69–87.

Serrani Azcurra, DJ. Traducción al español y validación de una batería ejecutiva (BE25) y su versión abreviada (ABE12) para la detección de disfunción ejecutiva en demencias. *Neurología*. 2013; 28(8):457-76.

Sherman, E, Tan, J, and Hrabok, M. *A Compendium of Neuropsychological Tests: Fundamentals of Neuropsychological Assessment and Test Reviews for Clinical Practice*. Oxford University Press, Oxford, UK: 2023.

Sierra Sanjurjo, N, Montañes, P, Sierra Matamoros, FA, et al. Estimating intelligence in Spanish: Regression equations with the Word Accentuation Test and demographic variables in Latin America. *Applied Neuropsychology Adult*. 2015; 22: 252–61.

Smith, A. *Symbol Digit Modalities test*. Western Psychological Services, Los Angeles, CA, U.S.: 1973.

Smith, GP, and Burger, GK. Detection of malingering: Validation of the Structured Inventory of Malingered Symptomatology (SIMS). *Journal of the American Academy of Psychiatry and the Law*. 1997; 25: 183–9.

Sosa, AL, Albanese, E, Prince, M, et al. Population normative data for the 10/66 Dementia Research Group cognitive test battery from Latin America, India and China: A cross-sectional survey. *BMC Neurology*. 2009; 9: 48.

Spielberger, CD, Gonzalez-Reigosa, F, Martinez-Urrutia, A, et al. Development of the Spanish edition of the state-trait anxiety inventory. *Interamerican Journal of Psychology*. 1971; 5(3-4), 145-158.

Spitzer, RL, Kroenke, K, Williams, JB, et al. A brief measure for assessing generalized anxiety disorder: The GAD-7. *Archives of Internal Medicine*. 2006; 166: 1092–7.

Storey, JE, Rowland, JT, Basic, D, et al. The Rowland Universal Dementia Assessment Scale (RUDAS): A multicultural cognitive assessment scale. *International Psychogeriatrics*. 2004; 16: 13–31.

Strauss, E, Sherman, EMS, and Spreen, O. A compendium of neuropsychological tests: Administration, norms, and commentary, 3rd ed. Oxford University Press: New York, NY, U.S.: 2006.

Strutt, AM, Ayanegui, IG, Scott, BM, et al. Influence of socio-demographic characteristics on DRS-2 performance in Spanish-speaking older adults. *Archives of Clinical Neuropsychology*. 2012; 27: 545–56.

Strutt, AM, Scott, BM, Shrestha, S, et al. The Rey 15-item memory test and Spanish-speaking older adults. *The Clinical Neuropsychologist*. 2011; 25: 1253–65.

Stucky, K, Kirkwood, M, Donders, J, et al. *Clinical Neuropsychology Study Guide and Board Review*. Oxford University Press, New York, NY, U.S.: 2020.

Suarez, PA, Diaz-Santos, M, Marquine, MJ, et al. Demographically adjusted norms for the Trail Making Test in native Spanish speakers: Results from the neuropsychological norms for the U.S.-Mexico border region in Spanish (NP-NUMBRS) project. *The Clinical Neuropsychologist*. 2021; 35: 308–23.

Suen, HK, Greenspan, S. Serious problems with the Mexican norms for the WAIS-III when assessing mental retardation in capital cases. *Applied Neuropsychology*. 2009; 16: 214–22.

Teunisse, S, Derix, MM, van Crevel, H. Assessing the severity of dementia. Patient and caregiver. *Archives of Neurology*. 1991, 48: 274–7.

Thurstone, LL. *Primary Mental Abilities*. University of Chicago Press, Chicago, IL, U.S.: 1938.

Tombaugh, T, Kozak, J and Rees, L. Normative Data Stratified by Age and Education for Two Measures of Verbal Fluency FAS and Animal Naming. *Archives of Clinical Neuropsychology*. 1999; 14: 167–77.

Torralva, T, Roca, M, Gleichgerrcht, E, et al. Validation of the Spanish Version of the Addenbrooke's Cognitive Examination-Revised (ACE-R). *Neurología*. 2011; 26: 351–6.

Torres, VL, Vila-Castelar, C, Bocanegra, Y, et al. Normative data stratified by age and education for a Spanish neuropsychological test battery: Results from the Colombian Alzheimer's prevention initiative registry. *Applied Neuropsychology Adult*. 2021; 28: 230–44.

Tropp, LR, Erkut, S, Coll, CG, et al. Psychological acculturation: Development of a new measure for Puerto Ricans on the U.S. mainland. *Educational and Psychological Measurement*. 1999; 59: 351–67.

Troyer, AK. Normative data for clustering and switching on verbal fluency tasks. *Journal of Clinical and Experimental Neuropsychology*. 2000; 22: 370–78.

Vasquez, PM, Tarraf, W, Li, Y, et al. Concordance between self-reported medical diagnosis of mild cognitive impairment/dementia and neurocognitive function among middle-aged and older Hispanic/Latino adults: Results from the Hispanic Community Health Study/Study of Latinos (HCHS/SOL) and the Study of Latinos-Investigation of Neurocognitive Aging (SOL-INCA). *Journal of Alzheimer's Disease*. 2022; 88: 45–55.

Veiga, BM, and Ordi, HG. Detección de simulación en estrés postraumático y depresión (Detection of malingering in post-traumatic stress & depression). *Revista de Psicología y Educación*. 2007; 6(1), 35-52.

Vercammen, KA, McClain, AC, Tucker, KL, et al. The association between baseline acculturation level and 5-year change in adiposity among Puerto Ricans living on the mainland United States. *Preventive Medicine Reports*. 2019; 13: 314–20.

Vila-Castelar, C, Munoz, N, Papp, KV, et al. The Latin American Spanish version of the Face-Name Associative Memory Exam is sensitive to cognitive and pathological changes in preclinical autosomal dominant Alzheimer's disease. *Alzheimer's Research & Therapy*. 2020; 12 (1): 104.

Vila-Castelar, C, Papp, KV, Amariglio, RE, et al. Validation of the Latin American Spanish version of the face-name associative memory exam in a Colombian Sample. *The Clinical Neuropsychologist*. 2020; 34: 1–12.

Warrington, EK, and James, M. *The Visual Object and Space Perception Battery*. Thames Valley Test Company: Edmunds, Suffolk: 1991.

Wechsler, D. *Wechsler Memory Scale-Revised*. Psychological Corporation, New York, NY, U.S.: 1987. *Escala Wechsler de Inteligencia para Adultos* – III. Manual Moderno: Mexico City, Mexico: 2003. *Escala de Inteligencia Wechsler para Adultos* – Tercera Edición (EIWA-III). Pearson: San Antonio, TX, U.S.: 2008. WAIS-III: *Escala de Inteligencia Wechsler para Adultos-III*. T.E.A. Ediciones, Madrid, Spain: 1999.

Weintraub, S, Besser, L, Dodge, HH, et al. Version 3 of the Alzheimer Disease Centers Neuropsychological Test Battery in the Uniform Data Set (UDS). *Alzheimer Disease and Associated Disorders*. 2018; 32: 10–17.

Weintraub, S, Dikmen, SS, Heaton, RK, et al. The cognition battery of the NIH toolbox for assessment of neurological and behavioral function: Validation in an adult sample. *Journal of the International Neuropsychological Society*. 2014; 20: 567–78.

Weintraub, S, Randolph, C, Bain, L, et al. Is cognitive decline measurable in preclinical Alzheimer's disease?. *Alzheimer's & Dementia*. 2017; 13: 322–23.

Wells, FL. Sex differences in the tapping test: An interpretation. University of Illinois Press, Urbana, IL, U.S.: 1909.

Widows, MR, Smith, GP, Ordi, HG, et al. Sims: *Inventario Estructurado de Simulación de Síntomas: Manual*. Tea ediciones, Madrid, Spain: 2009.

Woodcock, RW, McGrew, KS, Mather, *N. Woodcock-Johnson III Tests of Cognitive Abilities and Tests of Achievement* (3rd ed.)*. Rolling Meadows, IL, U.S.: Riverside Publishing: 2001.

Yesavage, JA, and Sheikh, JI. Geriatric Depression Scale (GDS): Recent evidence and development of a shorter version. *Clinical Gerontologist*. 1986; 5: 165–73.

Zea, MC, Asner-Self, KK, Birman, D, et al. The Abbreviated Multidimensional Acculturation Scale: Empirical validation with two Latino/Latina samples. *Cultural Diversity & Ethnic Minority Psychology*. 2003; 9: 107–26.

Zepeda, MUP, Guerrero, JAR, Carrasco, OR, et al. 2008. P3-038: Validation of the neuropsychiatric inventory questionnaire in a group of Mexican patients with dementia. *Alzheimer's & Dementia*. 2008; 4: T527–T28.

Zubicaray, G, and Ashton, R. Nelson's (1976) Modified card sorting test: A review. *The Clinical Neuropsychologist*. 1996; 10: 245–54.

Zuno Reyes, A, Trejo, S, and Matute, E. Linear and nonlinear effect of years of schooling, sex, and age on the CERAD-MX and complementary tasks in a Mexican sample: A cross-sectional Study. *Archives of Clinical Neuropsychology*. 2023; 38: 962–75.

Table: Description of Tests Norms by Domains

Test	Articles	Geographic Area/Countries	Sample Size	Age (Mean and Range)	Education (Mean and Range)	Gender % Female	Bilingual (Y/N)	Test Publicly Available (Y/N)	Where to Access
BRIEF COGNITIVE SCREENING MEASURES									
Mini-Mental State Examination (MMSE)	O'Bryant et al, 2018	Texas/Mexican American	412	>40	9.9 (SD 4.6)	73%	NR	N	
	Stricks et al, 1998	Northern Manhattan/ Dominican, Puerto Rican	996	Spanish 74.7 (SD 6.2)	Spanish: 6.1 (SD 4.2)	70%	NR	N	
	Marshall et al, 1997	Sacramento and Winters California/ Primarily Mexican American	753	71	8.5	56%	NR	N	
	Rosselli et al, 2000	Colombia	1506	>50	55.2% Had three or fewer years of schooling		NR	N	
MMSE-37	Contador et al, 2016	Spain	3777	65–97	11.9% Illiterate 41.7% Could read and write 31.9% Primary school 14.5 % Secondary or higher	56.4 %	NR	N	
Montreal Cognitive Assessment (MoCA)	Delgado et al, 2019	Chile	172	≥60 (73 ± 6)	11 ± 4; 17% ≤6 Years of education	53.1%	NR	Y	mocacognition.com
	Aguilar-Navarro et al, 2018	Mexico	168	76 ± 8.1	10.7 ± 5.2	80.4%	NR	Y	mocacognition.com
	Pereiro et al, 2017	Spain (Galicia)	563	50–97 (66.43 ± 11.16)	1–4, 5–8, 9–13 More than 13 years	57% Females	NR		

Test	Articles	Geographic Area/Countries	Sample Size	Age (Mean and Range)	Education (Mean and Range)	Gender % Female	Bilingual (Y/N)	Test Publicly Available (Y/N)	Where to Access
Evaluación Neuropsicológica Breve en Español (NEUROPSI)	Ostrosky-Solís et al, 2012	Mexico	950	53 (40–79)	8.23 (0–18)	78.7	NR	N	Pearson
Addenbrooke's Cognitive Examination-Revised/III	Torralva, 2012	Argentina	N = 127 (40 frontotemporal dementia; 46 AD and 40 CN	71,6 (6.9)	12.9 (4.5)	32 Males 95 Females	N	N	NA
	Matias-Guiu et al, 2015	Spain (Madrid, Barcelona y Oviedo)	273 Healthy subjects	70.10 (10.69) Years (range 50–94)	10.27 (5.44)	62.6% Females	N	N	NA
	Custodio et al, 2012	Peru	276	NR	NR	NR	N	N	NA
Mini-Cog	Carnero-Pardo et al, 2013	Spain (Madrid, Granada)	n = 307 176 Cognitive impairment	72.0 ± 10.1	<Elementary school = 50.8% >Elementary school – 49.2%	72% Females	N	N	NA
	Carnero-Pardo et al, 2022	Spain	581 (315 with CI)	63.8 (14.4) Years (range, 15–92)	<Elementary school = 27% >Elementary school = 73%	55.1% Women	N	N	NA
Six-Item Screener (SIS) from SOL-INCA	Breton et al, 2021	United States (Spanish Speaking Individuals from the Bronx, NY, Chicago, IL, Miami, FL, and San Diego, CA)	9309	56.5 (9.92)	11.0 Years (5.6)	54.5% Female	Y	N	NA

continued

Test	Articles	Geographic Area/Countries	Sample Size	Age (Mean and Range)	Education (Mean and Range)	Gender % Female	Bilingual (Y/N)	Test Publicly Available (Y/N)	Where to Access
GLOBAL COGNITIVE SCREENING MEASURES/NEUROPSYCHOLOGICAL BATTERIES									
Consortium to Establish a Registry for Alzheimer's Disease (CERAD)	Torres et al, 2019	Antioquia, Colombia	2673	32.94 (18–86)	8.89 (1–25)	56	NR		Contact author
Batería Neuropsicológica en Español	Artiola et al, 1999	Mexico, U.S. Border and Spain /Mexico and Spain	390	42.1 (SD 13.5)	9.6 (SD 6.1)	75	NR		Manual de Normas Y Procedimientos Para la Bateria Neuropsicologia—Lidia Artiola, Lidia Artiola I Fortuny—Google Books
NEUROPSI Atención y Memoria	Ostrosky-Solis et al, 2007	Mexico	521	6–85	0–3, 4–9, 10–22 Years				
Dementia Rating Scale (ST-DRS-2)	Strutt et al, 2012	Texas/Mexico, Argentina, El Salvador, Nicaragua, Venezuela, Puerto Rico, Guatemala, Peru, Honduras, Ecuador, Chile Uruguay, Dominican Republic and Cuba	157	65.3 (50–80)	13.6 (6–19)	61.8	NR	N	Not yet published
Neuropsychological Screening Battery for Hispanics (NeSBHIS)	Ponton et al, 1996	Los Angeles, CA/ Primarily Mexico, Central America	300	38.4 (16–75)	10.7 (1–20)	60	30% Bilingual 70% Monolingual		
The National Institute of Health Toolbox Cognition Battery	Weintrau et al, 2014; Casaletto et al, 2016; Gershon et al, 2020	Atlanta, Chicago – Oak Brook, Cincinnati, Columbus, Dallas, Los Angeles, Minneapolis, Philadelphia, Phoenix, and St. Louis	408 Neurologically healthy adults	Ages 18–85; M = 44.1, SD = 16.7	M Education = 10.7 Years, SD = 4.3	35% Male			

Test	Articles	Geographic Area/Countries	Sample Size	Age (Mean and Range)	Education (Mean and Range)	Gender % Female	Bilingual (Y/N)	Test Publicly Available (Y/N)	Where to Access
Repeatable Battery for the Assessment of Neuropsychological States (RBANS) – Form A*	Hall et al, 2018	Texas, New Mexico/ Mexican American	Spanish = 67	53 (40–79)	8.23 (0–18)	78.7	Not reported	N	Pearson
Spanish and English Neuropsychological Assessment Scales (SENAS)	Mungas et al, 2005	Sacramento Area, CA/Mexican	Total = 1374 Hispanic English = 357 Hispanic Spanish = 676 Whites = 341	70.9 (60–101)	Hispanic English 11 (0–21) Hispanic Spanish 5 (0–19) Whites = 14.1 (4–21)	46–60% Depending on group	41.3% Bilingual 1.7% Monolingual English, 27.6% Monolingual Spanish, 4.6% Pred English with some Spanish 24.8% Pred Spanish with some English	N	Contact authors of SENAS
Neuropsychological Assessment of the Spanish Speaker	Ardila, Roselli, and Puente, 1994	Colombia	N = 180 N = 360 N = 200	Three age groups five age ranges	Three education levels illiterate vs. professional		NR		Neuropsychological Evaluation of the Spanish Speaker| Springer Link
Rowland Universal Dementia Assessment Scale (RUDAS)	Coelho-Guimarães et al, 2021	Spain (Galicia)	150	76 (65–85+)	7 (0–16+)	59	NR		Validación del RUDAS como instrumento de cribado de población con demencia en atención primaria (nih.gov)

continued

Test	Articles	Geographic Area/Countries	Sample Size	Age (Mean and Range)	Education (Mean and Range)	Gender % Female	Bilingual (Y/N)	Test Publicly Available (Y/N)	Where to Access
INTELLECTUAL FUNCTIONING									
Wechsler Adult Intelligence Scale – Third Edition (WAIS-III)	Wechsler, 2001	Spain	1369	15–94 Years	Four education levels	51% Female	Yes	Pearson	https://www.pearsonassessments.com/en-us/Store/Professional-Assessments/Cognition-%26-Neuro/Escala-de-inteligencia-de-Wechsler-para-adultos-%7C-Cuarta-edici%C3%B3n%2C-Spain-Version-/p/P100022001?srsltid = AfmBOooa-y52dG8Wf-lw-yQ_hwwZwYa9I25uSdIKqzY0gm4dXFhosLBsH&utm_source = chatgpt.com
Escala de Inteligencia de Wechsler para Adultos, Tercera Edición WAIS-III: Mexico	Escobedo & Hollingworth, 2009; Weschler, 2003	Mexico	1000	16 ≥ 70	Two education levels (high school and higher or less than high school)	52% Female	NR	Manual Moderno, N	https://articulo.mercadolibre.com.mx/MLM-792418608-wais-iii-test-nuevo-y-completo-_JM?utm_source = chatgpt.com
Escala de Inteligencia de Wechsler para Adultos, Tercera Edición (EIWA-III) – Puerto Rico	Wechsler, 2008	Puerto Rico	330	16–64	0–16+	48% Female	NR	Pearson	https://euroamericanapr.com/producto/eiwa-iii-escala-de-inteligencia-de-wechsler-para-adultos-prueba-completa-espanol-c/?utm_source = chatgpt.com
Wechsler Adult Intelligence Scale – Fourth Edition (WAIS-IV)	Duggan et al, 2019 Weschler, 2012a, 2012b	Spain	1002	16–90	0–16+	52.3% Women	NR	Pearson	https://www.grupoquorum.com/libro/ver/815916-waisiv-manual-tecnico-y-de-interpretacion.html?utm_source = chatgpt.com

Test	Articles	Geographic Area/Countries	Sample Size	Age (Mean and Range)	Education (Mean and Range)	Gender % Female	Bilingual (Y/N)	Test Publicly Available (Y/N)	Where to Access
Wechsler Adult Intelligence Scale – Fourth Edition (WAIS-IV) *(continued)*	Duggan et al, 2019 Weschler, 2013	Chile	887	16–90	0–17+	50% Women	NR	Pearson, N	https://www.cedeti.cl/cedetest/tests-adultos/wais-iv/?utm_source = chatgpt.com
	Duggan et al, 2019 Weschler et al, 2016	Colombia	156	16–90	0–17+	50% Women	NR	Pearson, N	Not available
	Duggan et al, 2019 Wechsler, 2014	Mexico	1450	16–90	NR	51.9% Women	NR	Pearson, N	https://www.manualmoderno.com https://store.manualmoderno.com/escala-wechsler-de-inteligencia-para-adultos-91-300.html?utm_source = chatgpt.com
Reynolds Intellectual Assessment Scales (RIAS)	Reynolds & Kamphaus, 2009	European Spanish	2065	(3–94)	NR	NR	NR	N	Reynolds Intellectual Assessment Scales: Spanish with Norms|RIAS (parinc.com)
Batería III y IV Woodcock-Muñoz	Muñoz-Sandoval et al, 2005	Mexico, Central America, Spain	7416	(2–90)	(0–12+)	NR	NR	N	Batería IV Woodcock-Munoz (wpspublish.com)

continued

Test	Articles	Geographic Area/Countries	Sample Size	Age (Mean and Range)	Education (Mean and Range)	Gender % Female	Bilingual (Y/N)	Test Publicly Available (Y/N)	Where to Access
TESTS ASSESSING SPECIFIC DOMAINS									
PREMORBID LITERACY									
Word Accentuation Test (WAT)	Del Pino et al, 2019	Eight Geographical Locations in Spain	700	(18–86)	(0–12+)	56.4% Female	NR	Y	Demographically Calibrated Norms for Two Premorbid Intelligence Measures: The Word Accentuation Test and Pseudo-Words Reading Subtest – PMC (nih.gov)
Batería Woodcock-Muñoz III (Identificación de letras y palabras)	Muñoz-Sandoval, Woodcock, McGrew, and Mather, 2005	Mexico, Central America, Spain	7416	(2–90)	Kindergarten–12+	NR	NR	N	WPS Publish
ATTENTION									
Visuospatial Span, Corsi Test	Pena-Casanova et al, 2009	Spain: Castilla, Cataluña, Galicia, and the Basque Country	349	M = 64 (50 to 90 Years)	M = 10.4 (SD = 5.4) range = 0–20	59.6%	Y (Catalan, Galician, Basque)	Y	https://www.tetratrik.com/producto/cubos_corsi_wnv/
Digit Span Forward and Backward	Wechsler, 2013	Chile	887		0–18+				
		Colombia	156						
	Pena-Casanova et al, 2009	Spain: Castilla, Cataluña, Galicia, and the Basque Country	334	M = 64 (50 to 90 Years)	M = 10.4 (SD = 5.4) range = 0–20	59.6%	Y (Catalan, Galician, Basque)	Y	https://www.pearsonassessments.com/store/en/usd/p/P100022001.html?
	Wechsler, 2014	Mexico	1450	16–90					

Test	Articles	Geographic Area/Countries	Sample Size	Age (Mean and Range)	Education (Mean and Range)	Gender % Female	Bilingual (Y/N)	Test Publicly Available (Y/N)	Where to Access
WAIS-III and WAIS-IV – Letter-Number Sequencing	Rivera Mindt et al, 2021	California/Arizona	202	37.32 (19–60)	10.67 (0–20)	58.66	Y	Y	https://www.pearsonassessments.com/en-us/Store/Professional-Assessments/Cognition-%26-Neuro/Escala-de-inteligencia-de-Wechsler-para-Adultos-%7C-Tercera-Edicion/p/100000192?srsltid = AfmBOoqzlqfIvSsugCezHc2-PfGem4QQxDbW
	Peña-Casanova et al, 2009	Spain: Castilla, Cataluña, Galicia, and the Basque Country	356	64 (50–90)	M = 10.4 (SD = 5.4) (range = 0–20)	59.6%	Y (Catalan, Galician, Basque)	Y	https://www.pearsonassessments.com/store/en/usd/p/P100022001.html?
WAIS-R Arithmetic	Rivera Mindt et al, 2021	California/Arizona	183	37.1 (19–60)	10.67 (0–20)	58.66	Y	Y	https://www.pearsonassessments.com/en-us/Store/Professional-Assessments/Cognition-%26-Neuro/Escala-de-inteligencia-de-Wechsler-para-Adultos-%7C-Tercera-Edicion/p/100000192?srsltid = AfmBOoqzlqfIvSsugCezHc2-PfGem4QQxDbW
Paced Auditory Serial Addition Test (PASAT) – 50 and 200 (NP-NUMBRS)	Rivera Mindt et al, 2021	California/Arizona	251	37.32 (19–60)	10.67 (0–20)	58.66	NR	Y	PASAT form

continued

Test	Articles	Geographic Area/Countries	Sample Size	Age (Mean and Range)	Education (Mean and Range)	Gender % Female	Bilingual (Y/N)	Test Publicly Available (Y/N)	Where to Access
ATTENTION (continued)									
Brief Test of Attention	Arango-Lasprilla, 2015	Argentina, Bolivia, Chile, Cuba, El Salvador, Guatemala, Honduras, Mexico, Paraguay Peru, Puerto Rico	3977	18–95	Grouped 1–12 and 12 and over		NR		
Bells Test	Carrión et al, 2024	California, Connecticut, Florida, Indiana, New Jersey, Oregon, Virginia, and Wisconsin	245 Spanish-speaking adults	18–80 (41.1 ± 14.9)	15.1 ± 4.2	60.8%	Y	Y	
"A" Cancellation Test	Torres et al, 2021	Antioquia, Colombia	2673	32.94 (18–86)	8.89 (1–25)	56	NR	N	Ask authors
Number Span Test (UDSv3)	NIA Alzheimer's Disease Research Center	Mexico (41%) South American (22%) PR (11%) Central American (9.4) m Cuba (7%) Dominican (5.8%)	437	71.3 (50–94)	11.4 (0–20)	75.40	NR		
EXECUTIVE FUNCTIONING									
Trail Making Tests	Arango-Lasprilla et al, 2015	Argentina, Bolivia, Chile, Cuba, El Salvador, Guatemala, Honduras, Mexico, Paraguay Peru, Puerto Rico	3977	18–95	Grouped 1–12 and 12 and over		NR	Y	
	Peña-Casanova et al, 2009	Spain: Castilla, Cataluña, Galicia, and the Basque country	356	64 (50–90)	10.4 (0–20)	59.6	NR	Y	

Test	Articles	Geographic Area/Countries	Sample Size	Age (Mean and Range)	Education (Mean and Range)	Gender % Female	Bilingual (Y/N)	Test Publicly Available (Y/N)	Where to Access
Trail Making Tests *(continued)*	Rivera Mindt et al, 2021	Mexico	251	37.32 (19–60)	10.67 (0–20)	58.66	NR	Y	
	Torres et al, 2021	Colombia	2673	32.94 (18–86)	8.89 (1–25)	56	NR	Y	
	NIA Alzheimer's Disease Research Centers – UDSv3	Mexico (41%) South American (22%) PR (11%) Central American (9.4)m Cuba (7%) Dominican (5.8%)	437	71.3 (50–94)	11.4 (0–20)	75.40	NR	Y	Uniform Data Set version 3| National Alzheimer's Coordinating Center (naccdata.org)
	O'Bryant et al, 2018	Texas/Mexican American	412	40+	9.9		NR		
Symbol Digit Modalities Test (SDMT)	Arango-Lasprilla et al, 2015	Argentina, Bolivia, Chile, Cuba, El Salvador, Guatemala, Honduras, Mexico, Paraguay, Peru, Puerto Rico	3977	18–95	Grouped 1–12 and 12 and over		NR		
	Peña-Casanova et al, 2009	Spain: Castilla, Cataluña, Galicia, and the Basque country	356	64 (50–90)	10.4 (0–20)	59.6	NR		
Wisconsin Card Sorting Test (WCST-48)	Torres et al, 2021	Antioquia, Colombia	2673	32.94 (18–86)	8.89 (1–25)	56	NR		

continued

Test	Articles	Geographic Area/Countries	Sample Size	Age (Mean and Range)	Education (Mean and Range)	Gender % Female	Bilingual (Y/N)	Test Publicly Available (Y/N)	Where to Access
EXECUTIVE FUNCTIONING (continued)									
Wisconsin Card Sorting Test (WCST-64)	Arango-Lasprilla, 2015	11 Latin-American Countries: Argentina, Bolivia, Chile, Cuba, El Salvador, Guatemala, Honduras, Mexico, Paraguay Peru, Puerto Rico	3977	18–95	Grouped 1–12 and 12 and over		NR		
Verbal Fluency: Controlled Oral Word Association Test (COWAT) (P,M,R,F,A,S) and Semantic Fluency	Arango-Lasprilla, 2015	11 Latin-American Countries: Argentina, Bolivia, Chile, Cuba, El Salvador, Guatemala, Honduras, Mexico, Paraguay Peru, Puerto Rico	3977	18–95	Grouped 1–12 and 12 and over		NR		
	Rivera Mindt et al, 2021	Mexico	246	37.32 (19–60)	10.67 (0–20)	58.66	NR		
	Torres et al, 2021	Antioquia, Colombia	2673	32.94 (18–86)	8.89 (1–25)	56	NR		
	O'Bryant et al, 2018	Texas/Mexican American	412	40+	9.9		NR		
	NIA Alzheimer's Disease Research Center	Mexico (41%) South American (22%) PR (11%) Central American (9.4) Cuba (7%) Dominican (5.8%)	437	71.3 (50–94)	11.4 (0–20)	75.40	NR		

Test	Articles	Geographic Area/Countries	Sample Size	Age (Mean and Range)	Education (Mean and Range)	Gender % Female	Bilingual (Y/N)	Test Publicly Available (Y/N)	Where to Access
Stroop Color-Word Interference Test	Arango-Lasprilla, 2015	11 Latin-American Countries: Argentina, Bolivia, Chile, Cuba, El Salvador, Guatemala, Honduras, Mexico, Paraguay Peru, Puerto Rico	3977	18–95	Grouped 1–12 and 12 and over		NR		
LANGUAGE									
Boston Naming Test (BNT-60)	Olabarrieta-Landa and Rivera et al, 2015	11 Latin American Countries	3779	10–95					
	Peña-Casanova et al, 2009	Spain	340	50–94	<5, 6–7, 8–9, 10–11, 12–13, 14–15, 16 or >	59% Females			
BNT-30	Ponton et al, 1996								
Boston Naming Test (BNT-30, odd) (UDSv2)	NIA Alzheimer's Disease Research Center	Mexico, South American, Puerto Ric, Central American, Cuba, Dominican	437	71.3 (50–94)	11.4 (0–20)		NR	Y	Uniform Data Set version 3| National Alzheimer's Coordinating Center (naccdata.org)
Boston Naming Test (BNT-15)	Torres et al, 2021	Antioquia, Colombia	2673	32.94 (18–86)	8.89 (1–25)	56 Females	NR	N	Ask authors
	Olabarrieta-Landa and Rivera et al, 2015	Costa Rica	563	59–90					
	Fillenbaum, 2007	Part of the CERAD – California & Pennsylvania	88 CN controls and 140 AD patients	70.45 (9.6)	5.53 (4.43)	69.24 Females			

continued

Test	Articles	Geographic Area/Countries	Sample Size	Age (Mean and Range)	Education (Mean and Range)	Gender % Female	Bilingual (Y/N)	Test Publicly Available (Y/N)	Where to Access
LANGUAGE (continued)									
Texas Spanish Naming Test (TNT)	Marquez de la Plata et al, 2008	Dallas, Mexican-born	85 From Primary Care Clinics	65 or Older					
Multilingual Aphasia Examination	Rey & Benton, 1991	Cuba, Mexico and Puerto Rico		6–69			NR	N	Multilingual Aphasia Examination, 3rd Edition| MAE (parinc.com)
Multilingual Naming Test (MINT-32) (UDSv3)	NIA Alzheimer's Disease Research Center Marquine et al, 2023	Mexico, South American, Puerto Rico, Central American, Cuba, Dominican	437	71.3 (50–94)	11.4 (0–20)	75.40	NR	Y	Uniform Data Set version 3| National Alzheimer's Coordinating Center (naccdata.org)
Token Test – 36 items	Peña-Casanova et al, 2009	Spain	348	50–94					
	Rey & Benton, 1991	As part of the Spanish Multilingual Aphasia Examination (MAE) Standardization	234	18–70	<4 years, 5–7, 8–11, 12–15, 16+)			Y	Psychological Assessment Resources, Inc.
Token Test – 15 items	Julio-Ramos et al, 2024	Chile	210 Healthy adults and 197 stroke patients					Y	
Multilingual Aphasia Examination – 3rd Edition (MAE)	Rey et al, 1999	Cuban, Mexican and Puerto Rican	234	18–70	<4 Years, 5–7, 8–11, 12–15, 16+		NR	N	Psychological Assessment Resources, Inc.

Test	Articles	Geographic Area/Countries	Sample Size	Age (Mean and Range)	Education (Mean and Range)	Gender % Female	Bilingual (Y/N)	Test Publicly Available (Y/N)	Where to Access
VERBAL MEMORY									
Weschler Memory Scale IV – Escala de Memoria Weschler, Versión España IV	Wechsler, 2013	Census based sample from Spain	810	Range = 16–89 (no mean provided)	Based on census (sin estudios, primer, segundo, tercer grado)	54.2%	N	N	WMS-IV manual
Wechsler Memory Scale-Third Edition (WMS-III): Logical Memory	Campos-Magdalen et al, 2024	Madrid, Spain	736 for LM-I and 725 for LM-II community-dwelling adults	Range = 50–88	Categorical variable divided into ≤5 year, 6–11, 12–15, and ≥16 years	66%	N	N	https://doi.org/10.1037/pas0001292
Wechsler Memory Scale-Third Edition (WMS-III) Logical Memory	O'Bryant et al, 2018	Texas/Mexican American	653 Community-dwelling adults for memory measures	40+	Mean = 9.9 (no range provided)	73.4%	Y (participants chose language of testing) 51.7% Spanish speakers	N	https://doi.org/10.1080/87565641.2017.1401628
Wechsler Memory Scale-Fourth Edition (WMS-IV) Logical Memory	Brugulat-Serrat et al, 2021	Spain	248	Mean = 60.5 (50–70)	Mean = 13.6 (8–20)	61.7%	N	N	https://doi.org/10.3233/JAD-210640
Wechsler Memory Scale-Fourth Edition (WMS-IV) Verbal Paired Associates	Wechsler, 2013	Census based sample from Spain	810	16–89	Based on census (sin estudios, primer, segundo, tercer grado)	54.2%	N	N	WMS-IV manual
Craft Story	Marquine et al, 2023	Alzheimer's Disease Research Center in the U.S.	437	50–94					

continued

Test	Articles	Geographic Area/Countries	Sample Size	Age (Mean and Range)	Education (Mean and Range)	Gender % Female	Bilingual (Y/N)	Test Publicly Available (Y/N)	Where to Access
VERBAL MEMORY (continued)									
Spanish English Verbal Learning Test (SEVLT)	Gonzalez et al, 2001	Predominantly of Mexican ancestry (88.2%), in California	689	60 and Older (mean = 69.7)	Mean = 8.4	58.7%	Y	Y	https://doi.org/10.1017/S1355617701755026
Spanish English Verbal Learning Test (SEVLT)	Gonzalez and Mungas, 2002	Predominantly of Mexican ancestry (%), in California	1686	60 and Older (mean = 70.32)	Mean = 7.28	58.6%	Y	Y	https://doi.org/10.1076/clin.16.4.439.13908
Brief SEVLT (B-SEVLT)	Breton et al, 2021	Health Study/Study of Latinos (HCHS/SOL), a large, multi-site cohort Hispanic/Latino groups (Central American, Cuban, Dominican, Mexican American, Puerto Rican, and South American)	9309	45 and Older (mean = 56.5)	Mean = 11	54.5%	Y (86% Preferred Spanish)	Y	https://doi.org/10.1002/dad2.12260
Hopkins Verbal Learning Test Revised (HVLT-R)	Arango-Lasprilla 2015	Argentina, Bolivia, Chile, Cuba, El Salvador, Guatemala, Honduras, Mexico, Paraguay Peru, Puerto Rico	3972 Analytic sample	18–95	Grouped 1–12 and 12 and over	Varies by country	NR (all Spanish speakers)	N	Reach out to authors https://doi.org/10.3233/NRE-151286
	Cherner et al, 2007	U.S.-Mexico border (Arizona and California)	127	Mean = 37.5 (range = 20–55)	≤6 = 4.5 7–9 = 8.5 10–12 = 11.6 ≥13 = 15.6 (range = 0–20)	57.4%	N (only monolingual Spanish)	Reach out to authors	https://academic.oup.com/acn/article-abstract/22/3/343/2875?redirectedFrom = fulltext

Test	Articles	Geographic Area/Countries	Sample Size	Age (Mean and Range)	Education (Mean and Range)	Gender % Female	Bilingual (Y/N)	Test Publicly Available (Y/N)	Where to Access
Hopkins Verbal Learning Test Revised (HVLT-R) *(continued)*	Diaz-Santos et al, 202	U.S.-Mexico border (Arizona and California)	201	Varies per education band: ≤6: 40.3 7–10: 37.9 11–12: 35.3 ≥13: 37.8 range = 19–60	Varies per education band: ≤6: 4.6 7–10: 8.6 11–12: 11.8 ≥13: 15.9	Varies per education band: ≤6: 58.7% 7–10: 56.8% 11–12: 66.7% ≥13: 54.8%	All tested in Spanish (based on objective language dominance and preference) but testing was in Spanish only	?	https://doi.org/10.1080/13854046.2020.1861329
	Sáez-Atxukarro et al, 2021	Spain	700	Range = 18–90	Range = 0–25	56.4%	NR	?	https://doi.org/10.33588/rn.7202.2020412
Memory Capacity Test (MCT)	Torres et al, 2021	Antioquia, Colombia	2673	32.94 (18–86)	8.89 (1–25)	56	NR	N	Reach out to authors
The World Health Organization, University of California, Los Angeles, Auditory Verbal Learning Test	Arango-Lasprilla et al, 2024		245						
NEUROPSI – Atención y Memoría: Word List/Stories	Ostrosky-Solís et al, 2007	Mexican American	950	53 (40–79)	8.23 (0–18)	78.7	NR	N	Pearson
Spanish Verbal Selective Reminding Test	Campo et al, 2004	Spain	263	34 (18–59)	13.93 (6–13+)	141 Females	NR	Y	10.1076/1380–3395 (200004) 22:2;1–1;FT279

continued

Test	Articles	Geographic Area/Countries	Sample Size	Age (Mean and Range)	Education (Mean and Range)	Gender % Female	Bilingual (Y/N)	Test Publicly Available (Y/N)	Where to Access
VERBAL MEMORY (continued)									
The Free and Cued Selective Reminding Test (FCSRT)	Bonete-Lopez et al, 2020	Spain	96	65.7 (55–87)	11.39 (3–19)	67.7% Women	N	NR	
The Free and Cued Selective Reminding Test (FCSRT)	Labos et al, 2008	Argentina	239	57.02 (range not reported)	12.03 (range not reported)	127 F	N	NR	
The Free and Cued Selective Reminding Test (FCSRT)	Peña-Casanova et al, 2009	Spain	340	Mean not reported; inclusion 49+ (50–94)	Mean not reported; range from stratification groups: ≤5 to ≥16	59.71 Women	N	NR	
The Free and Cued Selective Reminding Test (FCSRT)	Mokri et al, 2013	Mexico	538	78.7 (range NR)	6.7 (range NR)	55.2% Women	NR (participants had to be fluent in Spanish)	NR	
CERAD Word List	Torres et al, 2021	Antioquia, Colombia	2673	32.94 (18–86)	8.89 (1–25)	56	NR	N	Reach out to authors
	O'Bryant et al, 2018	Texas/Mexican American	412	40+	9.9	73	NR	N	Consortium to Establish a Registry for Alzheimer's Disease (CERAD)|Duke Center for the Study of Aging and Human Development
CERAD Word List	Aguirre-Acevedo et al, 2007	Antioquia, Colombia	999	50–70+	1–12+	233	N	NR	
CERAD Word List	Henao et al, 2010	Medellin, Colombia	848	50–95; Whole sample: 64.4 (MCI: 72.19; AD: 69.3)	Whole sample: 8.9 (MCI: 8.6; AD: 6.3)	446 Total (MCI: 29F; AD: 122F)	N	NR	

Test	Articles	Geographic Area/Countries	Sample Size	Age (Mean and Range)	Education (Mean and Range)	Gender % Female	Bilingual (Y/N)	Test Publicly Available (Y/N)	Where to Access
CERAD Word List	Fillenbaum et al, 2006	Spanish-speakers from the USC and University Pennsylvania	330	Average age stratified by CDR groups at each site	Average education stratified by CDR groups at each site	Percent male reported by CDR group at each site	NR	NR	
CERAD Word List	Carrion-Baralt at al, 2009	Puerto Rico and controls from English-speakers from NY	PR: 81, NY: 62	90+ (PR: 92.82; NY: 92.75)	PR: 8.87; NY:15.76	PR: 57.3% F; NY: 64.5% F	NR; PR: Spanish-speaking; NY: English as first language	NR	
CERAD Word List	Sosa et al, 2009	Cuba, DR, Venezuela, Peru, Mexico, China, India	14967	Percent reported by age groups in each country, site and urban/rural	Percent reported by education groups in each country, site and urban/rural	Percent females reported in each site	NR	NR	
CERAD Word List	Guerrero-Berroa et al, 2016	Costa Rica, Puerto Rico	95	93.7 (90–102)	2.9 (0–6)	68.3% Females	NR	NR	
CERAD Word List	Zuno-Reyes et al, 2023	Mexico	392	38.75 (18–59)	10.42 (0–24) (figure also reports education range as 0–30)	50.25% Women	N	Y	
The Loewenstein-Acevedo Scales for Semantic Interference and Learning (LASSI-L)	Curiel Cid et al, 2020; Crocco et al, 2018; Loewenstein et al, 2016	South Florida – USA	224 Cognitively healthy adults	Aged 60–95, including English speakers, and 72 Spanish speakers stratified by age	11.9 years				
Face-Name Associative Memory Exam	Vila-Castelar et al, 2020	Colombia	59	50.31 (27–82)	9.02 (2–17)	71% Female	N	Y	Reach out to authors

continued

Test	Articles	Geographic Area/Countries	Sample Size	Age (Mean and Range)	Education (Mean and Range)	Gender % Female	Bilingual (Y/N)	Test Publicly Available (Y/N)	Where to Access
VISUAL MEMORY									
Brief Visuospatial Memory Test – Revised (BVMT-R) (NP-NUMBRS)	Rivera Mindt et al, 2021	California/Arizona	202	37.32 (19–60)	10.67 (0–20)	58.66	NR	N	Reach out to authors
Batería Neuropsicológica en Español (BNE) – Memoria Visual	Artiola Fortuny et al, 1999	Madrid and the U.S.-Mexico border	390 (205 from Madrid and 185 from the U.S.-Mexico border)	U.S.-Mexico border 42.2; Spain 36.3; range: (19–73)	U.S.-Mexico border 9.6; Spain 12.7; range: (0–20)	U.S.-Mexico border 75; Spain 56	Y U.S.-Mexico: 24%; Spain: 12%	N	Purchase: https://www.baterianeuropsicologica.com/price
NEUROPSI – Attention and Memory	Ostrosky et al, 2007	Mexico (Mexico City, Colima, Guadalajara, Zacatecas)	521	Range: (6–85); Total sample age means not reported (reported only by stratified groups)	Range: (0–22) Total sample education mean not reported (reported only by stratified groups)	NR	N	N	Pearson
Wechsler Memory Scale-Third Edition (WMS-III)	O'Bryant et al, 2018	Texas/Mexican American	412	40+	9.9	73	NR	N	Pearson
Rey–Osterrieth Complex Figure	Arango-Lasprilla, 2015	Argentina, Bolivia, Chile, Cuba, El Salvador, Guatemala, Honduras, Mexico, Paraguay Peru, Puerto Rico	3977	18–95	Grouped 1–12 and 12 and over	NR	NR	N	Reach out to authors
	Torres et al, 2021	Antioquia, Colombia	2673	32.94 (18–86)	8.89 (1–25)	56	NR	N	Reach out to authors

Test	Articles	Geographic Area/Countries	Sample Size	Age (Mean and Range)	Education (Mean and Range)	Gender % Female	Bilingual (Y/N)	Test Publicly Available (Y/N)	Where to Access
VISUOSPATIAL CONSTRUCTIONAL ABILITIES									
Rey–Osterrieth Complex Figure	Arango-Lasprilla, 2015	Argentina, Bolivia, Chile, Cuba, El Salvador, Guatemala, Honduras, Mexico, Paraguay Peru, Puerto Rico	3977	18–95	Grouped 1–12 and 12 and over	NR	NR	N	Rey Complex Figure Test and Recognition Trial|RCFT (parinc.com)
	Peña-Casanova et al, 2009	Spain: Castilian, Catalan, Galician, and Basque	356	64 (50–90)	10.4 (0–20)	59.6	NR	N	
	Torres et al, 2021	Antioquia, Colombia	2673	32.94 (18–86)	8.89 (1–25)	56	NR	N	
The NEUROPSI Semi-Complex Figure Test	Ostrosky-Solís et al, 2012	Mexico	950	53 (40–79)	8.23 (0–18)	78.7	NR	N	Pearson
Benson Figure Test	NIA Alzheimer's Disease Research Center	Mexico, South American, Puerto Rico, Central American, Cuba, Dominican	437	71.3 (50–94)	11.4 (0–20)	75.40	NR	Y	Uniform Data Set version 3| National Alzheimer's Coordinating Center (naccdata.org)
Block Design (WAIS-R)	Rivera Mindt et al, 2021	California/Arizona	181	37.32 (19–60)	10.67 (0–20)	58.66	NR	N	Pearson
Judgment of Line Orientation (JOLO)	Peña-Casanova et al, 2009	NEURONORMA – Spain	341	50–90	Total sample: 10.4 (0–20); JOLO paper does not list, has stratifications	59.6 Total sample	Y	N	Ask authors

continued

Test	Articles	Geographic Area/Countries	Sample Size	Age (Mean and Range)	Education (Mean and Range)	Gender % Female	Bilingual (Y/N)	Test Publicly Available (Y/N)	Where to Access
VISUOSPATIAL CONSTRUCTIONAL ABILITIES (continued)									
CERAD Constructional Praxis	Torres et al, 2021	Antioquia, Colombia	2673	32.94 (18–86)	8.89 (1–25)	56	NR	N	Ask authors
Visual Object and Space Perception Battery (VOSP	Calvo et al, 2013	NEURONORMA – Spain	341	50–90	Total sample: 10.4 (0–20); VOSP paper does not list, has stratifications	59.6 Total sample	Y	N	Ask authors
FINE MOTOR SKILLS									
Grooved Pegboard Test	Rivera Mindt et al, 2021	California, Arizona/ Mexico	254	37.32 (19–60)	10.67 (0–20)	58.66	NR	N	Grooved Pegboard™|Human Evaluation by Lafayette Instrument Company (lafayetteevaluation.com)
Finger Tapping Test	Rivera Mindt et al, 2021	California/Arizona/ Mexico	181	37.32 (19–60)	10.67 (0–20)	58.66	NR	N	Finger Tapping Test – Adults/ Older Children – The Neuropsychology Center
DEMENTIA STAGING SCALES									
CDR® Dementia Staging Instrument (CDR-FTLD NACC) (UDSv3)	NIA Alzheimer's Disease Research Center	Mexico, South American, Puerto Rico, Central American, Cuba, Dominican Republic	437	71.3 (50–94)	11.4 (0–20)	75.40	NR	Y	Uniform Data Set version 3| National Alzheimer's Coordinating Center (naccdata.org)

Test	Articles	Geographic Area/Countries	Sample Size	Age (Mean and Range)	Education (Mean and Range)	Gender % Female	Bilingual (Y/N)	Test Publicly Available (Y/N)	Where to Access
DIGITAL NEUROPSYCHOLOGICAL MEASURES									
LASSI-L Digitized Version	Curiel Cid et al, 2021; Curiel Cid et al, 2024	Miami, Florida USA	112 English- or Spanish-speaking adults	Over age 59	12% of LASSI-D participants having less than a high school education, 20% completing high school, 27% reporting some college, 22% being college graduates, and 18% holding advanced degrees				
NIH Toolbox Cognition Battery (NIHTB-CB)	Casaletto et al, 2016c	408 Neurologically healthy adults	Ages 18–85						
VALIDITY OF TEST PERFORMANCE									
Test of Memory Malingering (TOMM)	Arango-Lasprilla, 2015	Argentina, Bolivia, Chile, Cuba, El Salvador, Guatemala, Honduras, Mexico, Paraguay Peru, Puerto Rico	3977	18–95	Grouped 1–12 and 12 and over	NR	NR	N	Pearson
Structured Interview of Malingered Symptomatology (SIMS)	Widows et al, 2009	Spain	1005	31.9 (17–71)	NR	66.4	NR	N	PAR INC
Rey 15-Item Test	O'Bryant et al, 2018	Texas/Mexican American	412	40+	9.9	73	NR	N	

continued

Test	Articles	Geographic Area/Countries	Sample Size	Age (Mean and Range)	Education (Mean and Range)	Gender % Female	Bilingual (Y/N)	Test Publicly Available (Y/N)	Where to Access
FUNCTIONAL SCALES									
Alzheimer's Disease Co-Operative Study ADL Scale for Mild Cognitive Impairment (ADCS-ADL-MCI)	Galasko et al, 2005		145	72.3 ± 9.2	NR	66.2%	NR	N	DOMS: Function Measures & Tools – DCRC (dementiaresearch.org.au)
Alzheimer's Disease Co-Operative Study ADL Scale for Severe Impairment (ADCS-ADL-sev)	Custodio et al, 2022	Peru	276 Participants were classified into AD (n = 113), MCI (n = 68), and cognitively healthy controls (n = 95)	>60	≥4 years	NR	NR	N	Detailed assessment of activities of daily living in moderate to severe Alzheimer's disease|Journal of the International Neuropsychological Society|Cambridge Core
THE ACTIVITIES OF DAILY LIVING QUESTIONNAIRE									
The Functional Activity Questionnaire (FAQ)	Gonzalez et al, 2022	39 ADRCs	27,916 (1269 Hispanics)	71.39 ± 10.56	15.21 ± 10.56	64.8%	NR		
Everyday Cognition (ECog)	Aguilar-Navarro, Sanchez et al, 2023	Mexico	200	73.4 ± 8.1	11.5 ± 5.3	63%	NR		

Test	Articles	Geographic Area/Countries	Sample Size	Age (Mean and Range)	Education (Mean and Range)	Gender % Female	Bilingual (Y/N)	Test Publicly Available (Y/N)	Where to Access
PSYCHIATRIC INVENTORIES									
Brief Symptom Inventory-18 (BSI-18)	Andreu et al, 2008	Madrid, Spain	200	16–70 38.40	N/R	55%	N/R	N	Pearson
Generalized Anxiety Disorder-7 (GAD-7)	García-Campayo et al, 2010	Spain	212	47.6 19–85	Numerical range is not reported (only qualitative ranges)	73%	N	Y	
	Pagan-Torres et al, 2020	Puerto Rico	302	35.79	Numerical range is not reported (only qualitative ranges)	74%	N/R	Y	
	Mills et al, 2014	United States	436	N/R	N/R	N/R	Y	Y	
Geriatric Depression Scale (GDS-30)	De La Iglesia et al, 2002	Spain	249	74.3 (65–100)	65% Illiterate	67.5%	NR	Y	Uniform Data Set version 3| National Alzheimer's Coordinating Center (naccdata.org)
Geriatric Depression Scale (GDS-15 in comparison to GDS-5)	Lucas-Carrasco, 2012	Spain	91	79.2 (55–91)	Less than primary school (43.6%) Primary school and higher (56.2%)	64.8%	N	Y	
Geriatric Depression Scale (GDS-15 in comparison to GDS-5)	Bugallo-Carrera et al, 2001	Spain	573	70.09 (50–80+)	0–4 years (13%) 5–8 years (45.2%) 9–13 years (24.1%) 13+ years (17.8%)	62.6%	NR	Y	
Geriatric Depression Scale (GDS-30)	Fernández-San Martín et al, 2002	Madrid, Spain	218	65–80	Illiterate to secondary studies	63.5%	N/R	Y	

continued

Test	Articles	Geographic Area/Countries	Sample Size	Age (Mean and Range)	Education (Mean and Range)	Gender % Female	Bilingual (Y/N)	Test Publicly Available (Y/N)	Where to Access
PSYCHIATRIC INVENTORIES (continued)									
Geriatric Depression Scale (GDS-15)	Baker and Espino, 1997	United States	41	74 (60–99)	N/R	44%	N/R	Y	
Geriatric Depression Scale – Telephone (GDS-T)	Carrera et al, 2001	Argentina	252	71.7	50% High school or college education	66%	NR	Y – GDS 30	
Geriatric Anxiety Inventory (GAI)	Marquez-Gonzalez et al, 2012	Spain	302	71.68	11.3	75.5%	NR		APA
Symptom Checklist-90-R (SCL-90)	De las Cuevas et al, 1991	Spain	570	18–74	NR	52.5%	NR	N	Pearson
Patient Health Questionnaire-9	Rosario-Hernández et al, 2023	Puerto Rico	969	21–30, 31–50, 51+	Average education = 15	55%	NR	Y	https://med.stanford.edu/content/dam/sm/ppc/documents/DBP/PHQ-9_bilingual.pdf
	Merz et al, 2011	United States	479	18–80	Some college education (40%)	100%	Y	Y	
Beck Depression Inventory-II (BDI-II)	Sanz, Perdigon, and Vasquez, 2003	Spain	470	18–29, 30–44, 45–59, 60 Years and older	No studies to specialization	52%	N	N	Pearson
	Penley, Wiebe, and Nwos, 2003	United States	122	62.5 (24–88)	NR	41%	Y-some	N	
	Rodriguez-Gomez, Davilla-Martinez, and Collazo-Rodriguez, 2006	Puerto Rico	410	75.6	8.3 (3.8–12.8)	77%	NR	N	

Test	Articles	Geographic Area/Countries	Sample Size	Age (Mean and Range)	Education (Mean and Range)	Gender % Female	Bilingual (Y/N)	Test Publicly Available (Y/N)	Where to Access
Beck Anxiety Inventory (BAI)	Magan et al, 2008	Spain	249	37 (18–78)	No education to university	52%	N	N	Pearson
	Blasquez et al, 2020	Mexico	1245	36 (18–73)	0–29	59%	N		
	Morejon et al, 2014	Spain	918	36.69 (15–74)	Incomplete primary school (2.6%) Primary school (4.9%) Secondary school (20.6%) Non-compulsory high school (33.2%) College (18.4%) Graduate school (13.1%)	62.4%	N		
State and Trait Anxiety Inventory (STAI) – Reduced	Fernández-Blázquez et al, 2015	Spain	489	74.34	10	62.09%	N	N	
Short Spanish Adaptation of State and Trait Anxiety Inventory (STAI)	Buela-Casal and Guillén-Riquelme, 2017	Spain	1157	29.73 (18–69)	NR	59.89	NR	N	

continued

Test	Articles	Geographic Area/Countries	Sample Size	Age (Mean and Range)	Education (Mean and Range)	Gender % Female	Bilingual (Y/N)	Test Publicly Available (Y/N)	Where to Access
BEHAVIORAL INVENTORIES									
Neuropsychiatric Inventory Questionnaire (NPI-Q) (UDSv3)	NIA Alzheimer's Disease Research Center	Mexico, South America, Puerto Rico, Central America, Cuba, Dominican Republic	437	71.3 (50–94)	11.4 (0–20)	75.40	NR	Y	Uniform Data Set version 3| National Alzheimer's Coordinating Center (naccdata.org)
Social Observer Behavior Checklist (SBOCL) (FTLD-NACC)	NIA Alzheimer's Disease Research Center	NR	NR	NR	NR	NR	NR	Y	FTLD Module version 3| National Alzheimer's Coordinating Center (naccdata.org)
Executive Interview 25 (EXIT 25) (TMAANS)	O'Bryant et al, 2018	Texas/Mexican American	412	40+	9.9	73	NR	N	Pearson
Behavioral Inhibition Scale (BIS; FTLD-NACC)	NIA Alzheimer's Disease Research Center	NR	NR	NR	NR	NR	NR	Y	FTLD Module version 3| National Alzheimer's Coordinating Center (naccdata.org)
Interpersonal Reactivity Index (IRI; FTLD-NACC)	NIA Alzheimer's Disease Research Center	NR	NR	NR	NR	NR	NR	Y	FTLD Module version 3| National Alzheimer's Coordinating Center (naccdata.org)
Revised Self-Monitoring Scale (RSMS; FTLD-NACC)	NIA Alzheimer's Disease Research Center	NR	NR	NR	NR	NR	NR	Y	FTLD Module version 3| National Alzheimer's Coordinating Center (naccdata.org)
Mild Behavioral Impairment Checklist (MBI-C)		Santiago de Compostela, Spain	111	>50	NR	NR	NR	N	N/A

Test	Articles	Geographic Area/Countries	Sample Size	Age (Mean and Range)	Education (Mean and Range)	Gender % Female	Bilingual (Y/N)	Test Publicly Available (Y/N)	Where to Access
ASSESSMENT OF CULTURAL VARIABLES									
BILINGUALISM									
Linguistic History Questionnaire (CLS) (UDSv3)	NIA Alzheimer's Disease Research Center	Mexico, South America, Puerto Rico, Central America, Cuba, Dominican Republic	437	71.3 (50–94)	11.4 (0–20)	75.40	NR	Y	Uniform Data Set version 3| National Alzheimer's Coordinating Center (naccdata.org)
NP-NUMBRS Fluency Ratio (FAS/PMR)	Rivera Mindt et al, 2021	California/Arizona	254	37.32 (19–60)	10.67 (0–20)	58.66	NR	N	Reach out to authors
Language Experience and Proficiency Questionnaire (LEAP-Q)	Kaushanskaya, Blumenfeld, and Marian, 2019	Chicago	Study 1: 52 bilinguals Study 2: 50 bilinguals	Study 1: M = 27.29 years Study 2: M = 26.7 years	Study 1: M = 18.04 years of education SE = 2.62 (range = 15–27 years) Study 2: M = 16 years of education, SE = 2.5 (range = 11–22 years)	Study 1: 55.7% Study 2: 62%	NR	Y	LEAP-Questionnaire « Bilingualism and Psycholinguistics Research Laboratory (northwestern.edu)
ACCULTURATION									
Short Acculturation Scale for Hispanics (SASH)	Marin et al, 1987	San Francisco, CA	Hispanics (Primarily Mexican Americans, Cubans and Central Americans): n = 363 Non-Hispanic whites: n = 228	Hispanics: 31.2 years Non-Hispanic whites: 38.8	Hispanics: 12.3 years Non-Hispanic whites: 14.7	Hispanics: 62% Non-Hispanic whites: 57%	NR	Y	Development of a Short Acculturation Scale for Hispanics (sagepub.com)

continued

Test	Articles	Geographic Area/Countries	Sample Size	Age (Mean and Range)	Education (Mean and Range)	Gender % Female	Bilingual (Y/N)	Test Publicly Available (Y/N)	Where to Access
ACCULTURATION (continued)									
The Acculturation Scale for Mexican Americans (ARSMA)	Cuellar et al, 1995	South Texas	Mexican Americans: N = 379	NR	The average was 1 to 2 years of college	48%	Y	Y	ARSMA-II-Scala 1 (5) Muchísimo o casi todo el tiempo (4) Mucho o ... (yumpu.com)
Scale of Ethnic Experience (SEE)	Malcarne et al, 2006	California	Study 2 Group 1: n = 638 students Group 2: n = 1727 Study 3: n = 228 students Study 4: n = 265 students	Study 2 Group 1: M = 20.12 years, SD = 4.35 Group 2: M = 18.73, SD = 2.38	Participants were all college students from the San Diego State University	Study 2 Group 1: 60% women Group 2: 66% women	Y	Y	https://pmc.ncbi.nlm.nih.gov/articles/PMC9869708/
Psychological Acculturation Scale	Tropp et al, 1999	Boston and Puerto Rico	Study 1: n = 156 Latino/Latina college students Study 2: n = 90 Latino/Latina community members	Study 1: M = 23.49 years Study 2: M = 38.92 years	N/A	Study 1: 72% Study 2: 60% Study 3: (adolescents group): 52%	N	Y	
Abbreviated Multidimensional Acculturation Scale Hispanic-American Version (AMAS)	Zea, Asner-Self, Birman, and Buki, 2003	Mid-Atlantic Region of the U.S.	N = 246	M = 46.64	Study 1: Unknown Study 2: M = 10.54 years	Study 1: 60% women Study 2: 52% women	NR	Y	AMAS-ZABBpaper.pdf

Test	Articles	Geographic Area/Countries	Sample Size	Age (Mean and Range)	Education (Mean and Range)	Gender % Female	Bilingual (Y/N)	Test Publicly Available (Y/N)	Where to Access
Sabogal Familism Scale	Sabogal et al, 1987 and Campos et al, 2019	San Francisco, CA; Miami, FL Sabogal et al, (1987) San Diego, CA; Bronx, NY; Chicago, IL; and Miami, FL Campos et al, (2019)	Sabogal et al, 1987: N = 679; Mexicans: n = 164 Cubans: n = 99 Central Americans: n = 145 Non-Hispanics: n = 27 Campos et al, 2019: n = 5313	Sabogal et al, 1987 Mexicans: M = 30.8 Cubans: M = 40.8 Central Americans: M = 30.2 Non-Hispanics: M = 38.8 Campos et al, 2019: M = 46.64	Sabogal et al, 1987 Mexicans: M = 11.5 Cubans: M = 12.6 Central Americans: M = 11.9 Non-Hispanics: M = 14.7 Campos et al, 2019: Education was reported on an ordinal scale: the education level of the sample ranged from less than high school to more than high school	Sabogal et al, 1987: Mexicans: 62.5% Cubans: M = 60% Central Americans: 66% Non-Hispanics: 57% Campos et al, 2019: 61.70%	Y	Y	Familism Scale|Measures Library (miami.edu)
Hispanic Stress Inventory and Hispanic Stress	Cavazos-Rehg et al, 2006 and Cervantes et al, 1991	Los Angeles	N = 493 U.S.-born: n = 188 Immigrants: n = 305	Total: M = 23.2, SD = 6.9 U.S.-born: M = 21.6 years Immigrants: M = 24.3 years	Total: M = 12.9, SD = 13.4 U.S.-born: M = 12.9 years Immigrants M = 13 years	Total: 48.3% U.S.-born: 58.5% Immigrants: 42%	Y	Y	Hispanic Stress Inventory

NR = Not Reported

Made in the USA
Monee, IL
12 September 2026

62980083R00105